THE MIGHTY FORK

HEALING YOUR MIND AND BODY WITH FOOD

By Miranda Sherman

ELECTRIC MOON PUBLISHING

The Mighty Fork: Healing Your Mind and Body With Food

eBook ISBN: 978-1-943027-06-4
Paperback ISBN: 978-1-943027-05-7

Published by Electric Moon Publishing
Papillion, NE 68046
www.emoonpublishing.com

Printed in the United States of America

Ordering information for print editions:
Special discounts are available on quantity purchases by corporations, associations, and others. For details, contact the Electric Moon Publishing website at the address above.

Design and production: Electric Moon Publishing Creative Services
Cover design/Interior design: Alyssa Busse

ELECTRIC
MOON
PUBLISHING

DISCLAIMER

This book is in no way designed to replace your medical doctor or offer you medical advice. Please use your best judgment in proceeding with any changes that you make to your diet and please consult a medical doctor before stopping any prescription medication.

"When God prepares to do something wonderful, he begins with difficulty. When he plans to do something very wonderful, he begins with impossibility."
-Unknown

DEDICATION

I'd like to thank the many people who have helped me on my healing journey along the way. This book and my own healing would not have been possible without their invaluable support, coaching, encouragement, commitment, and love.

To my husband Roger, my son Reid, my mom Dorothy, and dad Bill, my sister Joy, and her husband Randy, my brother Daniel, my brother Grant, and his wife Angela, my many friends who sat with me and held my hand along the way and asked nothing of me, my extended family, the Weston A. Price Foundation, including my local chapter in Colorado Springs, Colorado, and my healing group in Omaha, Nebraska. My gratitude cannot be expressed in words.

6

TABLE OF CONTENTS

PROLOGUE

If you've picked up this book, chances are that you or someone you love is struggling. That struggle comes in many forms. For some, the struggle is physical illness. For others, the struggle might be mental or emotional issues.

The message of this book is to give you a sense of hope you may have never felt before. Struggles and challenges in any form can become wonderful and amazing blessings if you let them. God can do his mightiest work through our greatest weaknesses. How do I know? Here's my story.

INTRODUCTION

The idea of healing with food is not a new one. There's nothing new under the sun. We absolutely know that food can heal us. It can also harm us. When you go to the grocery store and you see food in boxes, what do you think? The majority of these boxed foods aren't really food because the nutrients in most of these "foods" are dead.

The difference between living food and dead food is that living food retains its vital nutrients; vital nutrients are the elements that are necessary for sustaining life. For example, when you consume a carrot, you know it is a living plant. When you eat a steak, you know it originated from a cow. Yet, when you eat a chili cheese flavored cracker, where did its ingredients come from? Is there any real chili or cheese in that cracker? If not, what was used to create the chili cheese? Chances are, it was someone in a lab coat conjuring up a new chemical formula with a blend of proprietary substances that can be patented to "taste" like chili cheese. That is my definition of a dead food.

Whether you are buying organic boxes, or just regular boxes, that food is not alive. By definition, boxed food is processed food. Processed food has been rendered inert or unable to rot. Digestion is the process in which the body breaks down and absorbs nutrients. If the product begins as "dead food," there are no nutrients for you to absorb. Not only are nutrients absent from these processed foods, but your body has to work to break down the chemical components that are there. You get no benefit from the food; only the sensation of eating. I have learned after being really sick, that my body craves and desperately needs living food to be healthy.

Once upon a time, I heard something profound from an author/educator named Kristin Urdiales. Her message was that our bodies need real nutrients that come from real food. Real food is necessary for the body to heal and function optionally. Not fake food. Not food-like substances. Not just eating to make the hunger go away. Real, nutrient rich, vitamin packed food.

What have you eaten today? Did it come from a box? Did any of your meals or snacks contain something other than sugar, wheat, and chemicals? Did you eat a banana or a green bean? What kind of meat did you eat? Do you know where your eggs came from? For most of us, we don't have a good answer to any of these questions. In these pages, you'll learn what to eat, how to eat it, and why you're eating it.

A lot has changed for me over the years, including my health. I now feel better than I've ever felt in my entire life (and I just hit the big four-two this year.). Anyone can do this. You can do this. It's radical. It's simple. And it's all about food.

SECTION 1: FOOD MEDICINE

CHAPTER 1

Eating to Heal

In the years before I discovered Healing Foods, I took twenty vitamin pills a day. I had transitioned to eating mostly organic foods and ate very little gluten or wheat, but I continued to eat processed foods. It was organic food to be sure, but it certainly wasn't living food. I thought I was doing great, but I still wasn't feeling great. My own health symptoms continued with autoimmune struggles, anxiety and depression, and thyroid and hormone issues. I had to drag my body through each day and I knew this wasn't God's best for me.

Kristin Urdiales was the first person to introduce me to the idea that food really can heal you. I stopped taking all vitamin pills that day and my real healing began. Sometimes I will say, tongue in cheek, "I have food allergies," when they offer me processed food. But the truth is, I just can't eat dead food anymore. I say I am "allergic" to toxic additives that I don't need in my body. What my body desperately needs is nutrition.

What I do know is this; your body is a machine. A machine needs fuel to run properly. If you put water in a gas tank, it won't run. The tank will be full, but not full of what it really needs. If you put vitamin supplements in your body machine, it still won't run. You need fuel; fantastic "nature made it perfect" fuel. If you start really putting the best authentic food you can find into your body (a.k.a. fuel), your “machine” will knock your socks off.

Feed your body what it really needs and you’ll feel fantastic. I feel so good that it should be illegal. Is it challenging to eat this way? Yes. The world has moved to dead food, making real food hard to find. But with just a little forethought and planning, it really doesn’t have to be out of reach. I’m no Cordon Bleu chef, but I do know how to make good nutritious food from dynamite ingredients. As Julia Childs reminds us, use the best ingredients you can find, and your cooking will taste great.

"...you are the only person who has sole custody of your life. Your particular life. Your entire life ... Not just the life of your mind, but the life of your heart."

-Anna Quindlen

Here are my tips and tricks to simplify your life in the kitchen and to nourish yourself and your family with easy meals every day of the year. Not only that, but this will help to restore the life God meant for you to lead. Whether you've never felt that great or you're trying to recover from physical and health challenges, I've learned that eating the right foods in the right way will start you on the path to your real healing, real energy, and real life.

THE TAKEAWAY

FOOD IS MEDICINE. FOOD CAN HEAL YOU IF YOU'RE EATING THE RIGHT THINGS.

CHAPTER 2

Health Can Be Restored

The first place to begin is, of course, at the beginning. The start of any journey begins with the first step. Healing the damage you have done to your body is a great place to start.

If the concept of "food as medicine" is a new one, then you are asking yourself, "What kind of food should I eat?" Which of the thousands of diets will you follow? Caveman, juicing, protein only, or calorie-counters? A million people are telling you what you should (and shouldn't) eat. Let me simplify it for you. If God made it, you can eat it. If you made it from scratch, using good ingredients (God-made-ingredients), you can eat it. Be wary of anything else. What kind of food is "God food"? In keeping with my philosophy of keeping things simple, we will look at meat, dairy, eggs, fruits, and vegetables and the best ways to source these.

MEAT

Meat contains vital proteins for your body, amino acids (see the amino acid section in Chapter 3), and B vitamins. Meat needs to come from a holistic rancher who cares about the soils, the grasses, the animals, and the health benefit to you, the consumer. Then you should look at the field—the place where your beef came from before it made its way to your table. You need to see for yourself how the animal was raised. Not only will this ensure that great quality grass went into your beef (grass that is rich in nutrients), but you will also be connected and respectful of your meat.

All meats should be grass-fed and grass-finished. Avoid corn-finished meat (particularly beef) if you can. Corn is a great way to fatten an animal a few months before that animal is processed. It does bulk up the animal and gives it a great flavor. After all, corn is converted into sugar in a cow's body (and in your body, too). Fattening cows on corn in the final months before slaughter is a relatively new practice in the history of the world. It is not healthy for us or the cow.

Animals, as nature intended, are designed to be out grazing on pasture. This includes pork, chicken, beef, lamb, buffalo, turkey, etc. Good healthy grass (that is not chemically sprayed) is where the vitamins are located. Grass is packed full of nutrients. Sadly, humans cannot get the B vitamins we so desperately need on our own simply by eating grass. We need another animal to eat it, and when we eat them, we get B vitamins through these animals. It's not really the grass in which the B vitamins are located. It's the dirt. Animals, when they graze, chew up chunks of soil and dirt. I'm not willing to do that myself quite yet. That is, eat dirt. I've heard some folks are doing it over in Japan, but I'm not the "let's eat dirt" kind of girl. So the animal gets the B vitamins and then I get the vitamins by eating that animal (and enjoying a nice steak or hamburger rather than a bowl of dirt).

Please know that I am very respectful and grateful to animals and to the fact that they give up their lives for my benefit. I want to know my cow, my pig, and my chicken. Anytime an animal is "processed," it is a big deal. I don't take high quality meat for granted and I would encourage you to do the same. Your cow had a face and a name. This is not "disgusting," but a reflection of God's beauty. Please honor that animal by being aware of how it was raised, and eat that meat with enjoyment and the satisfaction that comes from really being nourished.

> "Let food be thy medicine, and let thy medicine be food."
>
> -Hippocrates

If you are a vegetarian and don't choose to incorporate meat into your diet, you can eat dirt and get all of the B vitamins you need for health. Some ancient cultures in South America were vegetarians and did get all of their nutrients this way. If you're not willing to eat dirt, or eat animals that eat dirt, then you will be B-vitamin deficient.

"Why can't I just take a pill?" you might be thinking. Do you know what B vitamin supplements are made of? I took them for quite a few years and felt worse until I investigated their ingredients. Most B vitamins are made of tar.

Let's take for example, vitamin B1. Coal tar is a commonly used substance in the manufacturing of synthetic B1 vitamin pills. Most often, a crystalline yellow coal tar that is derived from a fossil fuel (Andrews, 2014). The next step is for the manufacturer to add hydrochloric acid and then moisture. Fermented, heated, cooled, and pressed into shapes, a synthetic version of B1 is complete. It will be dried and tested, of course, and then appear on shelves everywhere as a fantastic supplement.

Now don't get me wrong, there are some stellar supplement manufacturers that use excellent ingredients. I have found that for a very deficient person, sometimes you need supplementation to bring your vitamin levels up. But try food as your first resort. Include a wide variety of foods rich in vitamins and nutrients before starting supplementation.

Let's look at the food sources of B1 (thiamine). You can find great levels of thiamine in brewer's yeast, sunflower seeds, and pine nuts. When I think about sitting down to enjoy a lovely snack that includes sunflower seeds, that sound tasty. But a big bowl of yellow crystalline coal tar? Blech.

Sourcing your food, and knowing your farmer can

feel overwhelming. How much more difficult is it then to source your vitamins? I'd have to travel to the plant, observe where they are procuring all the ingredients, watch the process, and then determine whether or not I am confident with how that supplement is made. Why would I do that when I could just do an online search for "foods containing the highest amount of B1" and then eat and enjoy, obtaining all the thiamine I need?

There's another catch, too. We as humans think we're absolutely brilliant and know everything there is to know. We've always thought we had everything figured out. Seven hundred years ago, when scientists swore that the world was flat and one would fall off of the edge if we traveled too far, they were sure this was true. We still think we're brilliant. And humans have done amazing things to be sure. But I think most scientists will agree that there are nutrients in the universe that we just haven't identified. We might think we need B1 or thiamine, but just maybe we need an undiscovered nutrient that is often found with B1-containing foods (like a yet to be discovered B26 perhaps?) Or maybe an undiscovered nutrient (like our imaginary B26) is the key to allowing our bodies to absorb B1? There's still so much we don't know about our amazingly complex bodies and our world.

In an isolated nutrient pill form, you will miss out on these undiscovered nutrients. You won't miss out when you are eating nature-made food because nature makes things perfectly. Do an online search for B1-rich foods and then cook yourself something with the best organic local ingredients you can find from these particular foods. Eat them daily until you feel great. If you need a blood test to confirm that it's working, by all means help yourself.

My husband needed to get a blood test for something this past year, and because of how we eat in our house, his doctor told him he had never seen a higher B12 level. My husband doesn't take vitamins. He just eats what I put in front of him. I have long been deficient in B12, so I'm always eating the highest B12 foods I can get, and my husband receives the benefits.

While we're on the subject, let's take a brief look at vitamin D. The majority of Americans are vitamin D deficient (Lite, 2009). This statistic holds true in spite of the fact that food manufacturers continue to "fortify" processed foods with vitamin D. A little known fact about vitamin D is that for proper absorption, vitamin A must be taken simultaneously (Mercola, 2012). Otherwise, your body can't utilize the vitamin D you have ingested or taken in supplement form. If you're taking a vitamin D supplement, you have to remember to take vitamin A as well as a healthy fat to be able to properly absorb vitamin D. God, however, did it perfectly. In foods that are rich in vitamin D naturally, vitamin A is almost always present in addition to a healthy fat. A great example of this is cod liver oil.

First and most difficult of all perhaps, you need to replace compromising foods. Replace these compromising foods that contain multitudes of chemicals and burden our bodies. We can let our digestion rest after a lifetime of ingesting non-food substances which add a burden to our bodies. Let's say goodbye (for now) to wheat, processed dairy (with only a few exceptions), food that comes in boxes (yes, organic too), and pre-cooked meats. Focus on fruits, vegetables, high quality meats, and superb dairy. Cheese (especially raw cheese) and eggs should be included on this list of nutrient-dense foods. These nutrients include a multitude of vitamins, minerals, proteins, amino acids, and all the building blocks we need for health.

Learn to make home-baked goods and switch from white sugar to maple syrup for sweetening. Maple syrup is a natural food. If you choose a brand that is truly "maple syrup," with no other additives, your body has a much easier time in digesting this ingredient. Honey would be another great sweetener to choose, since, once again, it is exactly as God made it.

Try to stick with soups that are full of rich broth, lentils, beans, and meats. Start cooking again. Yes, I am sending you back to the kitchen. Let's say goodbye to our microwave and use our stoves and ovens. It doesn't need to be complicated. Fry yourself an egg and cook up some bacon. Have an apple with good nut butter or slices of cheese (grass-fed, if you can get it). Think about whether your food is alive. Set a goal that 95% of the food you choose to eat will be nutrient–rich and truly think about feeding your body everyday with living foods.

MY STORY

Before I begin telling my story, I just want to say that I don't harbor bitterness toward anyone. I know from the bottom of my heart that my family and many healthcare practitioners did the best they knew to do with the information they had at the time. It was my journey to seek answers for myself. Equally important was for me to let go of the expectation that someone else was responsible for my health. They were not. I needed to wrestle with God over this issue just as Jacob wrestled with God in the desert until God blessed him. I have experienced some breaking, and some pain, but it has all ultimately been for my own good. This wasn't just a physical journey of healing, but a faith journey as well. I have been refined through this journey in a million little ways and that is exactly as it is supposed to be. I would love to see a world without pain, but the fact is, we wrestle with challenges to make us better and to draw us to the source of all healing, our great God.

My family owns a small family farm and ranch. It belonged to my grandparents, and then eventually my parents and aunt and uncle. It is a traditional farm. They grow and feed genetically modified organism, or GMO corn, to fatten the beef cattle before slaughter. They even sign an agreement each year with the genetically modified seed company, agreeing to their terms. It seems like I would have had access to the best food imaginable growing up. It was fresh and tasted great, but was laden with pesticides. I don't know if that contributed to my health issues or not, but I distinctly remember watching the crop duster spraying pesticides overhead as we played in the fields in the summertime.

A host of health-related symptoms began appearing in my youth, including rashes, swelling in my abdomen, and extreme fatigue. When I became seriously ill in my twenties, I was incapacitated with worry, anxiety, and depression. Since that time, I've discovered this can be a symptom of pesticides—specifically the pesticide glyphosate (Senf, Smith, 2016). This pesticide destroys the body's ability to use the amino acid L-tryptophan correctly. Symptoms of glyphosate poisoning can include: eating but never feeling full, gaining weight but always feeling hungry, depression, low energy, anxiety, and feelings of aggression (Senf, Smith, 2016). After studying the effects of glyphosate poisoning and looking back to my childhood, it makes you go "Hmmmm?"

FRUITS AND VEGETABLES

Real nutrients can be found in any kind of fruit or vegetable. Don't worry so much about how to eat it. Some diets are really hung up on whether it needs to be raw, steamed, or fried. Instead, the focus should be on eating as many vegetables as we can in a variety of ways. My personal goal is three cups of any kind of vegetable each day. Try to limit yourself to mainly low glycemic fruits such as raspberries, blueberries, strawberries, blackberries, and some tart green apples. "Glycemic" refers to the sugar content. Feel free to eat as much of these berries and low-glycemic fruits as you'd like. Fruits like pineapple, mango, peaches, and very sweet fruits, can cause problems because of their naturally high sugar content. Sugar is found to be a culprit in many health challenges. We'll talk more about that later.

Eating enough vegetables seems to be difficult for most people (I know it is for me). I can assure you from my own personal experience that as you learn to eat this way, your taste buds will change. You will change and gain a "refined" palate. Foods that simply didn't appeal to you before will seem like a treat. Personally, a special treat for me each day is a few mini-sweet peppers to crunch on or a bowl of blueberries. It might take a while for this to happen for you. Try not to worry in the meantime.

People often ask me if the produce I consume is organic. The answer is a resounding yes. So many chemical components go into commercially-processed fruits and vegetables. If I can limit my exposure to these in any way, I'm going to do it. These chemicals wreak havoc with our health. The fact is, if it isn't organically grown, it contains pesticide. Until only forty years ago, all crops were grown organically—for thousands of years. All the family gardens in Europe are "organic," and have always been this way.

Organic food is grown the traditional way without chemicals. Growing this way is natural and good for us. Europeans simply don't struggle as much as Americans with Type 2 diabetes or obesity. If you buy only organic fruits and veggies, I can promise you will see results in your health. I hope it won't take something drastic like a serious illness, before you choose all-organic produce.

I know that the cost of organic produce limits many from making this choice. In contrast, so many of us spend $35.00 or more on a bottle of vitamins or prescription drug copays. Let me assure you; you can get a large quantity of organic produce for $35.00.

You will be eliminating these types of chemicals from your diet if you choose organic produce over conventional produce: The benefits of switching to organic include:

- Eliminating up to sixteen pounds of chemicals per person annually (Loux, 2011).
- Stopping exposure to 600 active chemicals, few of which have been thoroughly tested for safety to humans and the environment, yet are legally allowed (Loux, 2011).
- 95% of American children test positive for having toxic pesticides in their urine. This will be eliminated.
- Children with the highest amounts of pesticides in their urine were 93% more likely to have attention deficit disorder, compared with children who have 0% pesticide in their urine (Butler, 2010). You can reduce the risk of ADD for your own children.
- Choosing organic foods reduces pollution due to run-off of these chemicals, packaging of the sprays, and truck exhaust by hauling these products all over the country.
- Choosing organic foods will support your local farms who offer these options.

MILK

I had never heard of raw milk before I began transforming my own eating habits. What was this mysterious substance called "Raw" milk. What was the difference between this and regular milk (which never appealed to me much)? Raw milk comes directly from the farm and is not pasteurized or homogenized. In fact, it isn't altered in any way. And it is delicious. The cream separates naturally. This is a wonderfully nutrient rich food to give your children as they grow, giving them adequate healthy fats for their brain and body needed specifically for their healthy growth. We fight over the milk each week in my own home because we love it so much.

Finding raw milk takes a little bit of effort. Each state has slightly different laws about purchasing raw milk which will require some detective work to find a raw milk producer in your area. Chances are, you'll either have to drive to the farm to pick it up each week, or meet your farmer at an agreed upon location. My family drinks two gallons a week. You'll want to find a farm with Brown Swiss, Jersey or Guernsey cows if you can. Their milk is higher in the good fats that you will want for healing. Jersey and Guernsey cows produce a kind of milk that is easier to digest for most people (Weston A. Price, 2015). Also important is knowing that your cow is eating grass almost all of the time; grass that has not been sprayed with pesticides. Good raw milk should taste spectacular too. The taste is based on what the cow is eating. (This is also true of beef you eat. The flavor of the meat is directly related to the kind of pasture your beef cow is eating).

You can find great books about the subject of raw milk at www.realmilk.com including raw milk producers and excellent books on the subject.

EGGS

Scrambled, fried, poached, frittata—eggs fixed in any way are great for you. If you believe you are allergic to eggs, I recommend that you try to buy your eggs from a better source. So many people believe they are allergic to eggs, but in reality, they are allergic to what their chicken is eating. Soy is one of the most common food allergies, and sadly, one of the most common ingredients in commercial chicken feed. Soy is a cheap filler—even in organic chicken feed.

My advice is that you try eggs from chickens that are fed very few grains, no soy, and allowed to forage as chickens should naturally do, eating bugs and grass. Ensure your farmer uses organic feed with no added soy fillers. Even better would be to get eggs from a farmer that allows their chickens to forage on pasture as nature intended. If you don't have a local farm to supply your eggs, please contact your local Weston A. Price chapter to find a list of farmers who are using great practices in your area. You'll find their contact information in the "Resources" section in the back of the book.

To test your sensitivity to eggs (and find out if you're truly allergic to a good quality egg), before going to bed, place a dab of egg yolk on your wrist, cover it with a

Band Aid, and sleep on it (literally). In the morning, take off the Band Aid and see if your skin where you placed the yolk is red or inflamed. If it is, you are allergic to eggs, my friend.

In my experience in working with many clients, I have never met anyone who is allergic to the yolk of an egg, if it is coming from a properly fed chicken. Some clients do show a positive allergic reaction to the white of the egg. This part of the egg can be difficult to digest.

"You cannot poison your body into health with drugs, chemo or radiation. Health can only be achieved with healthful living."

-T.C. Fry

Remember this mantra: "Pay your farmer or pay your doctor." I do live within a budget (a strict one), but the item we spend the most on in our budget is food—real food, and the best we can afford. If you can't afford the best of everything yet, work your way toward it. We all start out at the beautiful and trendy expensive big-name health food store and quickly realize that doing all our grocery shopping there isn't feasible. That's when you learn that local is usually fresher, tastes better, and is often a better price. If I go to the farm for pick up, I can get great deals. I have not personally found this to be true of farmers' markets. The trend I'm seeing lately at farmers' markets is gourmet food. Please understand that I do think we should support farmers' markets, but these are often an "extra" for my family. The bulk of my food comes directly from the farm, a buying club (a group of people who get together and buy many items in bulk at wholesale prices), or my local natural food store.

If you're more of a "let's go and see what they've got and then make something" sort of person, then farmers' markets might be the way to go. If you want very specific items, and if you're looking for the most economical way to eat nutrient-rich foods, then farmers' market might frustrate you.

When I shop at the local natural food store, my cart is not heaped like it used to be when I shopped at the big-box grocery stores. Now I am buying food without big packaging and air—this does take a little getting used to. I used to panic a little when I looked at my cart and it didn't seem like I had much in there but was still paying the same price as the big-box grocery store. I have come to realize there is more than enough food to last the week. Of course, invest in bulk items like rice, lentils, high quality butter, and meat. You can freeze pastured butter, cottage cheese, bacon, and lunch meat when it goes on sale.

A great place to start to find great sources of food is the Weston A. Price Foundation. This is an international organization that will teach you how to cook and prepare nutrient-rich foods that will nourish your body. You'll learn easy recipes and they'll even show you where to shop. Knowing which brands have optimal products is key, and the Weston A. Price Foundation has already done much of the homework for you. I want to emphasize that this is

What is "pastured"? Pastured also means grass-fed. It's when your chicken (or cow, or pig) is outdoors, foraging for grass and eating what these animals eat naturally. They are fed limited grain or no grain at all, but instead eat bugs (as in the case of the chicken) or green grass when in season. The highest amounts of B-vitamins come from pastured or grass-fed animals. When you can afford it, always buy grass-fed/pastured. Spend the most money on quality meat.

a journey and it took me over ten years to tweak my eating habits. When I found Weston A. Price and a group of people healing and growing and learning about wonderful food, I was really on my way. Forgive yourself as you go; these changes will not happen overnight. Start your journey with good intentions and keep on keeping on. You'll get there with persistence and dedication.

I have seen miraculous healing through food from such conditions as autoimmune, learning disabilities, hyperactivity, arthritis, and diabetes. So much is possible. I wish you could see what I've seen, not only in my own physical healing, but in the lives of people I've had the pleasure to know.

"So whether you eat or drink, or whatever you do, do it all for the glory of God."

-1 Corinthians 10:3 NLT

Healing always starts with God. God is the author of great health and he wants you to be healthy. Excellent health is our birthright. But the world we live in tries to take away all that is good. From the way we think to the way we literally nourish our bodies, the world wants to entice us with less than God's best. I truly believe from the bottom of my heart that you have to ask God where he wants you to start on this healing journey. Spend time every morning in the Bible, listening to God. He wants every part of you—including your physical health. I don't believe sickness comes from God, but I do know from my own experience that God can use whatever is going on in your life for his glory. Healing can happen for you, and prayer works. So pray, do your part, and watch God work.

SOME GUIDELINES TO FOLLOW ON THIS JOURNEY

What I'm here to teach you will primarily focus on food. Asking anyone to change their eating habits is a big step. I know, because I've done it, and I've been blessed to witness hundreds of others learning to change their own eating habits. It can be done. You will feel so amazing after just a couple of weeks that you'll always want to feel as vibrant and energetic. That's why I set out to write a book; to make this change as easy as possible.

Trust me, this isn't anything like a modern "dieting" book. I'm asking you to consider changing your lifestyle so you can rock this life and really live. I only eat food that tastes great. Of course I want to feel good, but that doesn't mean I'm going to eat something that doesn't taste wonderful, too. It has taken me many years to discover how to do this easily for myself and to allow spectacular real food to become a cornerstone of my family's life. The benefits of this lifestyle are too numerous to mention. You'll definitely spend more time in the kitchen, but, as a result, you'll be changing yourself and those who live with you or are within your circle of influence.

I never advocate forcing anyone to change, but this change happens naturally. When one person makes a change for the better, others are watching and they see the benefits for themselves. Never become a short order cook for those who live in your house and choose not to eat the way you eat. One friend of mine exhausts herself, cooking three different meals for the three different people who live in her household because she is trying to make this change. Stop—please.

Cook great food from the best ingredients you can find and afford and allow others to choose whether they want to eat with you or not. They are free to make another choice. That choice might involve them going to the grocery store themselves, but so be it. The only person you are truly responsible for is you. If you live with children, believe me, they will eat what you have in the house. Sure, you'll hear a lot of, "Don't we have anything to eat?" from your kids, but remind them that carrots, peppers, nuts, and an apple really are something to eat.

Of course, everyone is entitled to a choice. Another friend of mine eats a very clean diet, but her husband doesn't want to change his white-bread-eating ways. He has his groceries and she has hers. I know husbands who would like to eat better, but blame their wives because she is not ready to change her own eating habits. I stand behind you and say to you, you can do it. Don't wait for someone else to change or use this as an excuse to avoid doing what you are called to change in your own life. If you don't like what's being cooked, or you can see how this could be improved, take it upon yourself to start cooking. At the very least, for yourself. Decide on the healing foods that you absolutely need to restore your own body and then determine to cook these foods for you and others in your home if they are open to it. .Allow God to work on their hearts. Just do what you have been called to do.

The journey to eating nutrient-dense foods is so important, but we have yet to talk about one crucial fact. You are sick for a reason. Your health (or someone you love) has been compromised by processed foods, sugars, medications, stress, lifestyle, and emotions. Your stomach, small intestine, large intestine, and colon are being bombarded by a barrage of damaging things. This damage leads to gut permeability or "leaky gut." Think about your gut health in this way. It's like looking at a shag carpet. The shag of the carpet (called villi) is where most of your nutrient absorption takes place. If the shag is damaged by abuse from harmful substances, it cannot absorb all of those wonderful nutrients that it will then pass on to your body. This is why you need to repair your villi.

Leaky gut is the underlying cause of irritable bowel syndrome, almost all stomach issues, autoimmune disease, and much more. Autoimmune disease compromises a list of approximately 140 different diseases, including asthma, arthritis, multiple sclerosis, and fibromyalgia (Auto-ImmuneDiseaseList.com). True health falls apart in the stomach and intestines (Myers, 2014). The good news is, this is where health can be restored. By changing our food, we are changing our world; our internal world that is.

MY STORY

I have had intestinal problems for many years. As a child, I was exposed to the strep throat virus and subsequent round after round of antibiotics from a very young age. My mom tells a funny story about me "pretending" to take my medicine during one of these rounds. I was throwing the pills behind my bed and it didn't occur to my nine-year-old self that I would be found out when we moved to another city. Of course, once the bed was pulled away from the wall, my deception was discovered. I guess I knew, even then, that all of those antibiotics weren't good for me. Antibiotics can be a lifesaver and I'm so glad they exist, however, they kill good gut bacteria along with harmful bacteria (Kressor, 2012). Each person needs to understand the potential dangers of antibiotics and work very hard after any course of antibiotics to restore their gut biome.

Restoring the gut flora can be done, in part, through fermented foods, which are living probiotics. Bear in mind that it's so much harder to restore healthy gut bacteria than it is to maintain the good bacteria that you were probably born with (unless your mother had poor gut bacteria before you were born or if you were born through a C-section and weren't exposed to your mother's gut bacteria the usual

"When you're green inside, you're clean inside."

-Dr. Bernard Jensen

way). Use antibiotics when there are no other options. Having infectious strep throat was a sign that my body was out of balance, even at a young age.

Growing up, I exhibited all the classic symptoms of a compromised immune system; strep, allergies, and fatigue. These red flags indicate your body is not getting the nutrients it needs and the gut is not in great health. Gut health is a key component to immunity and needs to be restored when there is a weak immune system and that was certainly the case for me. What I needed was to feed my gut biome. Instead, rounds of antibiotics exacerbated an already bad situation, setting me up for serious illness in my adult life. There is no blame, but with age comes wisdom. I do often say "if I had only known," but the wisdome came from living through it.

THE TAKEAWAY

FOOD IS MEDICINE, BUT YOU NEED TO KNOW WHICH FOODS HEAL. EATING FOR HEALING ALSO LIES IN KNOWING HOW YOUR FOOD IS PRODUCED AND WHO IS PRODUCING IT.

CHAPTER 3

Holy Trinity of Foods #1: Sauerkraut

Have I convinced you to eat differently yet? Don't worry, I will. I'm getting ready to simplify it even more. You should begin your healing with three almost miraculous healing foods. For our purposes, we'll call them the Trinity. Start here and eat them daily. These are the foods that will be the foundation of your healing. In the following pages, I'll show you how to make "dosages" for yourself with this new kind of medicine called food. It's quite easy, so take my hand and here we go.

This is where you're going to start. I know it doesn't sound earth shattering, but it is. You need one raw, fermented food every day. Raw fermented foods provide billions of healthy bacteria to our gut, and, most importantly, help us to absorb what we eat. These foods also provide us with hydrochloric acid production so we can digest all of these wonderful foods. Hydrochloric acid is what our bodies use to break down food. Many of us simply don't have enough hydrochloric acid to do this job properly. If we eat the best food on the planet, but aren't absorbing any of it, then we have wasted our time. Sauerkraut is easy to make and the best ingredient for restoring your health. Home-

"One-quarter of what you eat keeps you alive. The other three-quarters keeps your doctor alive."

-from a Hieroglyph found in an ancient Egyptian tomb

made sauerkraut is even better. Check out my free YouTube video at

https://www.youtube.com/watch?v=9KBw0_vfbcw.

On a cutting board, remove and disable the two outer layers of leaves, then chop your entire head of cabbage finely. Throw away the core. Place your diced cabbage into a pan and add one tablespoon of salt per two pounds of cabbage. Massage your cabbage thoroughly until it looks shiny. Don't be afraid to really squeeze. Place the cabbage into your Fido jar and add brine (see recipe below) to cover. The liquid should end up about four inches above the cabbage.

Brine recipe: four cups of filtered water to cover cabbage, adding 1 tablespoon of quality salt. If you need more liquid to cover, add 1 more tablespoon salt to every 4 cups of water added. Pour over your diced cabbage and seal the Fido jar. Write on a piece of tape the date three weeks from today's date and stick it on your jar as a reminder of when your sauerkraut will be ready to eat.

Burp your jar (a.k.a. open the bail) and CO2 will cause a slight "pop." Do this every day. (Or, you can search on YouTube on "How to Adjust the Bale on a Fido jar" and follow the directions. If you adjust the bale, you won't need to burp it each day). Reseal your jar and allow it to sit in a cool dark place under a tea towel for three weeks. At the end of three weeks, place your sauerkraut into smaller glass jars and store them in the fridge for up to six months. The flavor will intensify over time.

Easy Sauerkraut Recipe

-1 head organic green cabbage (the organic allows for all the best bacteria to proliferate)
-1 Tbsp of quality salt per 4 cups of filtered water
-4-8 cups filtered water (to cover cabbage completely)
-large Fido jar (with bale adjusted)

What is a Fido jar? I tried many different methods of fermenting until I discovered the amazing Fido. It's the best I've found for fermentation because it prevents oxygen from getting into your ferment and creating mold. Fido is an Italian company that makes a sealable jar that has a strong enough glass to withstand the carbon dioxide buildup that naturally occurs in fermentation (this can be compared to the fizz in soda). The fizz is a natural result of the ferment and the reason why we need to "burp" our Fido jars every day—to release that gas. Otherwise, an explosion can occur. You can purchase Fido jars in my online store (see "Resources" in the back of the book) or at a kitchen store.

Consume four ounces of sauerkraut and juice, three times a day. Do this for at least three months to restore your gut ecology (that beautiful and complex group of healthy bacteria that live in your gut). Start slowly and see how your body adjusts. Some people don't notice too much right away, other than less bloating with meals perhaps, while others have a more challenging adjustment and have to ease into this with smaller doses. A sign that you need to go slower would be any kind of stomach upset, headache, etcetera, that would indicate changes as your body adjusts to this new healthy bacteria. In that case, you can start with one time daily and work up to a thrice daily dose.

Always eat sauerkraut when you eat any type of

protein because it will help with digestion. The sauerkraut juice is nicknamed "Liquid Gold" because it can be taken to stop upset stomach, heartburn, diarrhea, and nausea. I get phone calls and emails from those who've heard me speak about the benefits of amazing sauerkraut but didn't quite believe it. When they try it for themselves, they are amazed. It really does work.

If you absolutely cannot make your own sauerkraut, then you can purchase a less potent, although still effective, form at the health food store. The benefit of this amazing food is starting to hit the mainstream market and some forward-thinking companies are now producing amazing krauts. There are a few wonderful brands on the market. Just make sure that the brand you purchase is raw, organic, and fermented. If it isn't organic, then it has been sprayed with pesticides, which kills the beneficial bacteria on the cabbage, and the ferment will not proceed as it was intended. Refrigerate it at all times to preserve the living enzymes and beneficial bacteria (canned sauerkraut is not the same).

MY STORY

As a child, I contracted mononucleosis at the age of three. As I grew older, I suffered with severe eye allergies. These allergies were the catalyst for my parents taking me to Children's Hospital in Denver on a regular basis. The doctors there treated me with modern medicine's answer for a cure—steroids. Modern medicine's idea of healing is to suppress symptoms. Steroids are immune suppressors. They are trying to stop the body's response to illness rather than address the root cause.

As I grew older, I had mysterious aches, pains, and lack of energy. My family doctor told me over and over that there was nothing wrong with me and insinuated I was a hypochondriac—that it was all in my head. In truth, my upper arms ached so severely that I would wrap them tightly with ace bandages just to relieve the pain.

Knowing that I wasn't just making it up, my mother took me to National Jewish Hospital in Denver where I was officially diagnosed with chronic fatigue syndrome; in short, an autoimmune condition that really did not have a definitive cure. The hospital used me as a guinea pig and experimented on me with various treatments, such as multiple rounds of antibiotics, steroids of progressively stronger strength, cortisone (which is an alternate form of steroids) and prescriptions that I can't even name. None of it really helped.

When I was a child, as my birthdays approached, I would get so excited about my special day that this would land me on the couch. Apparently, my body couldn't handle even the good strain of getting excited. My body was working so hard just to keep me up and moving on a daily basis and I couldn't handle one more thing; even one more great thing. While everyone else celebrated, I laid there with no energy; not feeling well enough to get up and join them for my own party.

At age thirteen, after multiple infections and many rounds of antibiotics, I developed extreme stomach pain with extensive abdominal bloating. Again, the doctors said there wasn't anything wrong with me, even though at times I would have such severe stomach problems that I would have a bout of dry heaving and then need to take very strong Motrin before I could escape the pain. This continued on into my high school years, during which I became so exhausted that I would sleep in the backseat of my car at lunchtime.

When I was eighteen, I became an exchange student in Germany. They had very little processed food in Germany (and it was expensive), so we ate real nutrient-rich foods (not including all of the pastries I consumed, of course.) I felt the best I'd ever felt in my life. On my return to the States, my health started to go downhill again. I lived on a diet of Dr. Pepper and pizza in college and became very sick. Again, I had no energy, had pale skin, I bruised easily, my upper arms ached, I had horrible spider veins on my legs, and I was just plain exhausted.

I suffered heat exhaustion a couple of times in these years and a heart doctor prescribed a statin drug to keep me from passing out in the heat of summer. This was the straw that broke an already sick camel's back. Statins are common "drug muggers," a term coined by Susie Cohen, which are the primary culprits in blocking vitamin absorption and these statins did exactly that for me. Since the statin drug I was taking blocked essential B vitamins, I began to have horrible symptoms of anxiety, depression, confusion, and even suicidal thoughts on a prescription cocktail that has a well documented list of these side effects. Sadly, my doctor was unaware of these common side effects listed on the warning that accompanied each prescription and I trusted that he had all the answers. He told me I had to stay on these drugs for my heart. I was warned that if I stopped taking them, the consequences could be horrible.

For five years, I followed my doctor's advice and continued to damage my body with these drugs that I never needed to take in the first place. Statins not only blocked my B vitamin absorption, but they also disrupted my hormones (a challenge I continue to deal with to this day. This affects my female hormones and weight gain, in my current life). Combine a really poor diet and lots of stress, and my overall mental and physical health tumbled out of control.

With the stress I was under in my young working life, I managed to destroy my adrenal glands, too. When you have destroyed your adrenal glands, you know it because you can't even drag yourself off the couch you have such extreme exhaustion. Another symptom of adrenal burnout, as it's often referred to, is the inability to handle the tiniest amount of stress without feeling overwhelmed. This period in my middle twenties was one of the most difficult times of my life. When I married my wonderful military husband, we moved to another state where I lived far away from family, didn't have a support system, and was so mentally ill with fears that I was not functioning. My husband did his absolute best to care for me, in spite of his extremely challenging job in the Air Force.

The military moved us once again, but to a community where I found much more support and more forward thinking doctors and alternative health practitioners. Hiking, clean air, pure water, stress reduction, and healthier lifestyles all contributed to a time of improvement in my health journey. After being married for five years and feeling physically stable, my husband and I decided this would be a great time to have a child.

After I became pregnant with my son, my health again took a turn for the worse. At the beginning of my pregnancy, I was extremely healthy and felt great. I still wasn't eating anything with real nutrients, but I had lots of energy and was very happy. During my eighth month of pregnancy, when the baby takes so many nutrients from the mom, I was laid flat. I must have had just enough nutrients stored up in my body to get that far, but then my body and mind threw in the towel. Literally, I would sit in the corner and rock. My brain burned—not a headache—but burned. I was beyond exhausted and couldn't handle the tiniest amount of stress.

My husband traveled extensively during those years with his military service, so I turned to my sister and my mom. They took amazing care of me the best they could. Some days, it felt like a miracle just to survive the day. I began to hate clocks during that time because it seemed like time crawled and I felt so miserable. I lay in bed most days and it took all I had to take care of my baby and myself.

THE REAL DIAGNOSIS

Looking back, I now know what was going on in my mind and my body. I had a compromised gut microbiome—probably from birth (my mom's gut isn't too healthy). When I caught mononucleosis as a child, this set the stage for future autoimmune disease. If I had eaten the nutrients I needed, as well consumed probiotics to restore my gut, all my health challenges might have been avoided. As a teenager, after multiple rounds of antibiotics, I showed the classic signs of candida overgrowth—a fungus that populates aggressively in our intestinal tract when we disrupt the balance by overuse of antibiotics and a diet high in sugar. I now know that the pains in my arms were a lack of nutrients needed for healthy growth as well as energy for my mitochondria (in my cells—to function well). My poor cells were "running on empty."

Teenagers need lots of nutrients to develop properly. It's a time of massive growth. My own son grew more than six inches this past summer, so I've recently witnessed this event in my own house. Research reveals that the common American teenager subsists on foods that not only lack any kind of nutrients, but deplete the body of nutrients as it tries to break them down (Home Health, 2013). And to add insult to injury, many of these foods in our modern era are laden with toxins which are poisonous to the body. Is it any surprise when I say that there are no nutrients in fast food or soda? And, if your children are eating these foods, they are eating a poisonous non-food substance.

Growing pains and lots of infections (colds, the flu, etc.) are strong symptoms of a lack of nutrients. Consider feeding your family in a way that ministers to their hearts, minds, and bodies. Even though my own son has shot up six inches this past summer, he never complained of growing pains (like I did when I was his age). Although we've been very successful with his nutrition, I can't say the same about our success with getting him to clean his room.

AMINO ACIDS: VITAL TO MY CURE

The horrific statin drugs I was put on in my twenties were the final nail in the coffin, dooming me to poor health. These poisons left me with a lifelong challenge of needing to restore my amino acids. I discovered amino acid therapy many years ago from a book by Julia Ross called "The Mood Cure". This book is the definitive work on amino acid therapy and its benefits with anxiety and depression. Since I was suffering from both of these things, I was motivated to read her work.

Amino acids control everything in your body, from how your cells function, to your moods, and how your hormones operate (or don't). The nine essential amino acids cannot be made by the body, but must come from food. These include phenylalanine, valine, threonine, tryptophan, methionine, leucine, isoleucine, lysine, and histidine. L-tryptophan is one of many essential amino acids which will keep a person emotionally steady, sleeping well, and feeling satiated rather than hungry because it helps produce serotonin. These were my biggest challenges.

Combine that with a leaky gut that can't reproduce these amino acids as it normally does, and I had set the stage for a cataclysmic health even in my own life; not only with my physical health, but with my mental health, too. A person can't be emotionally stable without these key and essential amino acids. Unfortunately, my first attempts with amino acid therapy weren't successful because I wasn't working with a practitioner and taking good brands of amino acids (only some of the brands are effective, even though you will find a wide variety of companies to choose from at any vitamin retailer).

A diet cleanup was my prescription too. I continued to deplete my nutrients and my amino acids as long as I was eating processed food. This meant replacing all of the non-food items that I loved to subsist on (can we say mini-powdered donuts and yummy coffee drinks?) and letting go of processed foods and sugars. I have to admit; I might not have been motivated enough to make this change if I hadn't been as sick as I was.

For your information, there are also six vital amino acids that should also be consumed through diet: arginine, cysteine, glycine, glutamine, proline, and tyrosine—all of which are important to your health. The reason I'm taking the time to tell you about all of these amino acids is that if you aren't eating a diet rich in nutrients, you aren't getting any of these vital amino acids.

Let's look at a simple amino acid: tyrosine. Tyrosine is an incredible (but not essential) amino. If you have low energy, aren't focused, or can't get yourself moving in the morning, look no further than foods that will increase your tyrosine. Keep in mind that this isn't even one of the essential amino acids. Amino acids have such complex jobs that I can't do them justice by explaining all that they control in this book. I will say amino acid therapy was the key to my recovery. Cleaning up my diet, prayer, exercise, and neurofeedback (we'll talk more about neurofeedback later) were vital, but correcting my amino acids healed me. Please do seek out more research on this topic for yourself.

I have also benefited greatly from the knowledge and work of Trudy Scott. I highly recommend Trudy Scott's website www.antianxietyfoodsolution.com for much more information and for finding a wonderful practitioner who is knowledgeable in the intricacies of amino acid therapy.

Work with a practitioner who is very comfortable with the latest research that is available on amino acid therapy since dosages can be challenging. I worked with a lovely practitioner in Iowa, Laurie Hammer, who was able to help me navigate the subtle world of amino acids. The method of supplementing with amino acids is complex, and a knowledgeable practitioner is critically important. Hire a professional and don't try to figure this out on your own.

I'm back on the road to health after ten years of finding great information. The internet is a wealth of learning. You might go down some bunny trails and have to reverse course now and again, but there is so much out there to learn for free. In my own healing, I am 98 percent cured. I'll have to manage stress for the rest of my life, supplement with amino acid therapy when needed, maintain a clean diet as well as eat many fermented foods each day, but it is worth it. Ten years ago, I couldn't have imagined how great I would feel a decade later. Even though it took me ten years to heal, you can accomplish your own healing much more quickly. I've done much of the research for you, and provided many of the resources so you should have no trouble feeling huge improvement almost immediately.

THE TAKEAWAY

SAUERKRAUT AND SAUERKRAUT JUICE IS YOUR FIRST "PRESCRIPTION." CONSUME SAUERKRAUT THREE TIMES A DAY FOR THREE MONTHS TO RESTORE YOUR GUT BACTERIA AND HELP YOU TO DIGEST FOOD. ABSORBING NUTRIENTS BROKEN DOWN FROM YOUR FOOD IS ESSENTIAL TO GOOD HEALTH. SAUERKRAUT IS ONE OF THE KEYS TO ABSORPTION.

CHAPTER 4

Holy Trinity of Foods #2: Raw Milk Kefir

Raw milk is a true superfood. Raw milk healed me in a dramatic way. Raw milk kefir played a vital role in my healing. Kefir helps break down the proteins in milk so that they are easier to digest. If you thought yogurt was good for you and your gut health, kefir is 1,000 percent more healing. The word "kefir" means "feel good" in Russian. Kefir itself is believed to have originated in modern day Russia or Turkey, in the North Caucus Mountains. Cultures have been consuming this beverage because of its benefits for hundreds of years.

One legend tells us that kefir grains represented a family's wealth in ancient times in these mountains. Those precious grains were passed down from generation to generation. It was a common belief that if they shared the "magical properties" of these special grains, then the kefir would lose its power. Marco Polo mentioned kefir grains in his writings in his travels to the East. It wasn't until the end of the 19th century that kefir came to other places in the world and was scientifically studied (History, 2002).

A wide variety of nutrients exist in kefir, including but not limited to many essential amino acids, B vitamins, vitamin A, vitamin D, calcium, iron, magnesium, and a whole host of yeasts and probiotics. It is the most widely consumed fermented drink in Russia and Eastern Europe, and it is sold worldwide. Dairy kefir is consumable by those who are lactose intolerant because the fermentation process removes the lactose. Sadly, commercial varieties of kefir are made from pasteurized milk which has already had its healthy bacteria destroyed in the pasteurization process. You'll want to obtain kefir "starter" grains from a good source. I carry them on my website, or you can often pick them up at your local health food store.

Take your raw milk, or the best, non-homogenized and low temperature pasteurized organic milk, and add your living kefir grains to a glass quart jar. Mix this together gently by swirling. Cover the top of the jar with a coffee filter and a rubber band to hold the filter securely in place. Set your jar and mixture in a warm place on your counter. I tend to set mine on my stove, but not on the burner. I put it in the middle of the stove where the warmth of the other burners is felt, but the kefir isn't in any danger of cooking. Seventy-eight degrees is the ideal temperature for your kefir.

Leave the milk on the counter for twelve to eighteen hours. That's right; just leave the milk on the counter. It will turn naturally into a yogurt-like drinkable yogurt.

When your milk has "kefired," you will see the whey (or clear part of the milk) separate from the curd (or the white part of the milk). Once the mixture has thickened in your original jar, place a stainless steel mesh strainer over a large bowl and pour the mixture through. Here you will capture your kefir grains. They look like clumps of tapioca pudding and can vary from the size of rice grains, to the size of walnuts. These grains are living organisms (similar to bread yeasts).

You can put them gently into a new jar of milk and start the process over again. Gently stir the kefir that you have strained, pushing it through the strainer with a rubber spatula to give it an even consistency. Pour your kefir into a clean jar and keep refrigerated until you consume it all.

When I made my first batch of kefir, my husband thought I was crazy. We were already buying raw milk—gasp—non-pasteurized milk. Then, to make kefir, the plan was to leave that raw milk on the counter overnight. This did not seem very safe to either of us. Isn't that the way you get food poisoning? But I soldiered on because I had done the research on the benefits of this amazing drink. My husband recommended I take my first glass of kefir to the hospital down the street and drink it in the emergency room parking lot, just in case. I did drink that first batch (at home) and survived. I had to start slowly since those beneficial bacteria are real. The first time I consumed raw milk kefir, my body definitely felt it. Something was going on "down there" as my stomach gurgled. You might want to start with just a small amount the first few days as your body adjusts to these new bacteria and yeasts. Since then, I have consumed thousands of glasses of kefir and I am not only surviving, but I'm thriving.

My favorite way to use kefir is to take a four-ounce

"dose" in the morning, and then another four-ounce "dose" in the evening before bed. Kefir is such an amazing and complex protein, chock-full of beneficial bacteria. It can, in just one example, immediately covert into the amino acid tryptophan in your body, which then converts to serotonin and finally, to melatonin. I often drink it plain (always with sauerkraut, of course, to help absorb all of the nutrients and digest the lactose), but you can add a teaspoon of good organic maple syrup or make a fruit smoothie.

Don't blend the kefir. You don't want to break those complex protein structures. You can blend fruit and water together in the blender and then stir in your kefir.

I have seen autistic children calm immediately after having a dose of kefir. I have also witnessed people who have temper tantrums and night terrors cease after starting on kefir therapy. If you have discovered that you are lactose intolerant, try a small amount of kefir and see how you react. In the case of raw milk, lactose intolerance usually stems from a lack of lactase in your milk. Lactase is the substance that you need to break down lactose, and it is destroyed during the pasteurization process. The kefiring process removes the lactose in the fermentation.

Start looking for a raw milk producer while you are doing your sauerkraut therapy. Try to eat sauerkraut for at least four weeks before starting on raw milk kefir to prepare your digestive system with all those wonderful beneficial bacteria in the sauerkraut. Then your body will be able digest kefir properly. It also takes some time to find a good milk source. I was on a waiting list for three months for raw milk from the first farm where I obtained raw milk from Colorado. I needed to begin restoring my gut with sauerkraut and also to stop eating damaging processed foods in the meantime, so the timing worked beautifully.

Try drinking raw milk, even if you've had trouble with milk in the past. Raw milk is so very different than store-bought milk; it will surprise you. I struggled to digest store-bought milk for years (and didn't even like the taste, to be honest). My family believes raw milk is in a class of its own. The taste does take a little getting used to because it is so rich and creamy. It is full of good fats, and good fats are needed for every cell in your body to work properly; most importantly, for your brain to work properly!

Honestly, this can be a slight adjustment for most folks. If you find that raw cow's milk is still bothering you, try raw goat's milk, which is also available in most areas. Those who can't drink raw milk, often find that raw goat's milk is fine because there is less casein in goat's milk. Casein is the protein found in milk that can be difficult to digest.

MY STORY

Kefir was a key nutrient-rich food for me. When I started drinking raw milk, I felt like I had real energy for the first time in my life. It must have been the good fats, the proteins, and the whole package which gave me this fantastic energy, calmed me, and made me feel happy. Nothing satisfies like raw milk. You feel good when you drink it. I used to drag through my days. Raw milk was my energy restoration. And dosing with raw milk kefir as a medicine is incredible for our health restoration. Now, I have so much "get up and go" that it's ridiculous. I have more energy now at forty-two than I had when I was ten years old. What an amazing food.

THE TAKEAWAY

RAW MILK AND MILK KEFIR IS YOUR SECOND "PRESCRIPTION" AS A HEALING FOOD. CONSUME FOUR OUNCES IN THE MORNING, AND FOUR OUNCES BEFORE BED. KEFIR CALMS YOU, HELPS RESTORE YOUR HEALTHY GUT BACTERIA, AND AIDS YOU IN PRODUCING SOME KEY AMINO ACIDS, LIKE TRYPTOPHAN.

CHAPTER 5

Holy Trinity of Foods #3: Bone Broth (a.k.a. Jewish Penicillin)

Bone broth should be part of everyone's regular diet. Broth made from high quality bones is extremely healing to your gut. These broths rebuild mucosa (the slime that lets food move well in our systems and also protects our digestive tract lining), and heals villi (the small shag-rug like lining of our intestines that allow us to absorb nutrients). Our ability to absorb food well is often compromised when we unintentionally damage these villi. The villi are weakened by junk food, processed foods, antibiotics, and other pharmaceuticals. We should try to be constantly rebuilding our digestive system as this is the primary way we get healing foods into our body. You can be eating the best food on the planet, but it's all for nothing if you're not absorbing it well.

Bone broth is here to save the day. The nutrients in bone broth include calcium, potassium, magnesium, and zinc. These nutrients are found in high quality bones (high quality like those we discussed in the "Meat" section) and are then transferred into our healing broth. Chicken soup (old fashioned and made with bone broth) will cure what ails you.

"Chicken soup is known for its curative properties. And anyone who has ever been tucked away in bed, miserable with a stuffy nose, knows the comfort and power of the golden broth, dotted with tender vegetables and soft noodles. While it's a folk remedy for the ages, researchers are beginning to discover just why and how chicken soup heals.

Chicken soup's curative properties have been documented for several centuries. In the 10th century, the Persian physician Avicenna referenced the healing powers of chicken soup. Again, in the 12th century Egyptian Jewish physician Maimonides recommended chicken soup to aid in the recovery from respiratory illnesses drawing his sources from classical Greek text. However, Maimonides and Avicenna weren't the only healers to recommend chicken soup to convalescents; rather, chicken soup seems to pop up as a healing food across the globe. Bottom line: stick to good, old-fashioned and traditional chicken soup. It's inexpensive to make, delicious and healthy with its anti-inflammatory properties." It's not just an old wives' tale after all (Chicken Soup Cure, 2009).

If you are ill and/or recovering from physical damage from surgery, an accident, or just stress, bone broth is vital to healing. It is straightforward to make and can be used in a variety of ways. You should always have some on hand for cooking soups, rice, and anything that calls for broth.

HEALING BONE BROTH #1: CHICKEN

Chicken carcass (bones, skin, meat left on the bones—organic and pastured of course. First, roast the chicken and then use the remaining carcass to do the following. For roasting information, see "Simple Roast Chicken" recipe on page 77.)

Carcass stripped from roasted chicken
Drippings from your roasting pan
¼ cup good apple cider vinegar (like Bragg's or Mother's Brand)
Filtered water to cover

Place the entire carcass, skin, bones, or connective tissue from your pan and the carcass into a slow cooker. Add water to cover the bones and vinegar. Let this sit for thirty minutes, allowing the minerals in the bones to be imparted into your broth. Cook on a low simmer for two days.

Strain and place broth in glass jars (I use half-gallon glass Mason jars). Glass jars won't impart any "chemicals" into your healing broth mixture (Wellness Mama). Cool in the refrigerator and remove the fat from the top after it is cold and has hardened. Save this fat for sautéing vegetables. Use the broth in a variety of recipes or simply drink eight ounces each day, warmed on the stovetop (no microwaves here please. They will destroy all those good nutrients).

Getting used to the taste might take some time. I like to simmer eight ounces in a small saucepan with a small amount of peeled and sliced raw organic ginger root, one-fourth of a teaspoon of good salt, and one tablespoon of lemon juice. This makes a tasty treat and much more enjoyable to drink than plain broth. Bone Broth can be made from any leftover bones in a similar manner. Please consume or freeze your broth within one week.

HEALING BROTH #2: BEEF BROTH

Use a mixture of bones of pastured organic beef bones from your butcher. Try to get some lean bones (like rib) and some meaty bones (like the leg bone). Brown the bones in your cast-iron pan with butter, turning each bone after a few minutes. Place the browned bones into your Crock-Pot (or stock pot, if preferred), with salt and pepper to taste. Let the bones sit in a pot of cool water for thirty minutes with one-fourth of a cup of vinegar and cook on the low temperature setting for two days. Strain and cool the liquid in glass half-gallon jars (as opposed to plastic) in your refrigerator. Remove fat from the top after the liquid cools. Use your broth in a variety of recipes found in this book or drink plain.

I have found that I like to cook a bone-in roast, eat the meat for a couple of meals, and then cook the bones into a broth. This seems to make the price for a quality, pastured, organic roast more do-able if I know I'm getting at least five meals out of it. We can get three meals out of the meat from the roast and two additional meals out of the broth.

MY STORY

Bone broth has had some amazing results in my life. I don't want to add more burden to my already weakened adrenal glands (see the previous chapter describing Adrenal Burnout). I wasn't able to exercise for many years due to a lack of energy. After about five years of consistently drinking bone broth, I now exercise each day, feeling energetic and strong. My hair and nails are revitalized and healthy, and my skin looks amazing without the eczema or acne from my younger years. No longer do I suffer from blotchy skin, which was always the bane of my existence as a pale, blond-haired, blue-eyed girl. The prominent spider veins on my legs have disappeared almost entirely. I'm even considering wearing shorts this summer, which I haven't done for a decade. Broth and other nutrient-rich foods have imparted strength and energy to my body in a way I'd never experienced before. My skin is tighter, too. And unlike the other women in my family, I don't have gray hairs peeking out.

Bone broth isn't something that works overnight. I've been consistent for many years and slowly saw the results in my own life. You will too—just stick with it.

Now that you've started on your three healing foods, learning how to alter what you cook so that you are providing the best possible, most economic meals for your family and yourself will be your next priority. I have simplified the process for you by offering uncomplicated menu ideas that you can adapt to meet your needs. Many of these recipes incorporate healing foods. Others complement the healing foods that you will be eating. Let's dive in.

"In the giving [of ourselves] it becomes clear that we are chosen, blessed and broken not simply for our own sakes, but so that all we are about, all that we live, finds its final significance in its being lived for others."

-Henri Nouwen (Catholic priest)

THE TAKEAWAY

BONE BROTH CAN REALLY HEAL YOUR GUT LINING IN A WAY THAT NO OTHER FOOD CAN, BY PROVIDING A POWERFUL SET OF VITAL NUTRIENTS THAT YOUR BODY CRAVES. YOUR THIRD FOOD "PRESCRIPTION" FOR HEALING IS ONE EIGHT-OUNCE CUP OF BONE BROTH EVERY MORNING, WARMED ON THE STOVE, AND SEASONED TO YOUR PREFERENCE.

SECTION 2: EVERYDAY COOKING

CHAPTER 6:

Week One: Winner, Winner, Chicken Dinner

Many years ago, I heard someone say it's a good idea to have fourteen "go to" meal ideas for a working menu in your home. You can rotate meals so that by the time you make a dish again, you'll be OK with eating it. I do add variety, depending on the season. In the fall, I crave soups and casseroles with more starches. In the winter I want meat. During the spring and summer, I tend to yearn for salads and fish. Once in a while, I throw in a few fancy dishes, like fillet mignon or a Thanksgiving turkey, but my basic "go to" menu is largely the same.

MY "GO TO" LIST

Some tricks of the trade: I like to make double batches so I'll have leftovers and maybe some to freeze for a day when I only have the energy to reheat something.

The following is broken down by weeks. I stretch my meals to keep it easy and economical. My primary goal is to cook something complicated once a week and keep it simple as the week goes on, often using the ingredients I've cooked earlier in the week. I don't want to be in the kitchen all the time any more than you. I also love the side benefits of saving time and money.

Meal 1: Roast chicken (later to become chicken broth); suggested sides: baked potato, zucchini and squash fry

Meal 2: Green Salad with chicken, walnuts, cranberries, goat cheese, and honey mustard dressing

Meal 3: Bacon, eggs, and fruit salad

Meal 4: Chicken and brown rice with sweet and tangy green beans

Meal 5: Smoky paprika red lentil soup and Italian salad

Meal 6: Teriyaki chicken stir fry

Meal 7: Chicken and dumplings: one pot meal

WEEK ONE RECIPES

You'll need a Crock Pot, a roasting pan with a baking rack, a skillet (I use cast-iron), and the list of ingredients (see below). You'll also find the groceries you'll need for the week below.

You probably already have many of these ingredients on hand. If not, these can become your new staples. Try to keep spices, and items that you can buy in bulk, stocked in your pantry. When I started eating this way, I didn't have a stocked pantry, but I quickly learned to buy in bulk when I could. Bulk buy groups, such as Azure Standard and Frontier Organics, are great ways to get a lot for less cost. Finding a few other people who want to share an order will drop everyone's prices even more. Purchase in season when the price is the best and freeze as much as possible.

- **2 pastured organic whole chickens (direct from the farmer if you can get them)**
- **1 package red lentils (buy in the bulk section; that's the best price)**
- **1 small package Hungarian paprika (again, bulk section)**
- **brown rice**
- **1 package pastured bacon**
- **4-5 kinds of fruit that you like, assorted, and ½ pound of each (I recommend berries of any kind)**
- **1 dozen eggs (always local, organic, grass-fed, and soy-free is best; know your chicken, and know your farmer)**
- **1 bag organic carrots**
- **1 bag organic celery**
- **2-5 cloves garlic (depending on your preference)**
- **1 pound organic green beans (frozen or fresh)**
- **½ pound organic green peas (frozen or fresh)**
- **Organic broccoli head**
- **Butter (pastured)**
- **2-6 organic zucchini and squash (depending on how many people you are feeding and the size of your squash)**
- **1 potato per person in your family, or that you are**

feeding. Yellow, red, or purple potatoes please. Don't use white potatoes; they do not contain many nutrients in comparison. You can substitute a sweet potato if you prefer.

- **8 small red potatoes (for other recipes)**
- **2 heads lettuce (organic). My personal preference is romaine or red leaf, but buy what's on sale that week.**
- **Walnuts (raw). Make them "crispy nuts." See the recipe in the "Extras" section.**
- **Dried cherries or dried cranberries (no sugar added)**
- **8 ounces soft goat cheese or chevre**
- **Lemon juice**
- **Raw cheddar cheese**
- **Dill (fresh or from the spice rack)**
- **Assorted spices**
- **1 jar or can organic artichokes**
- **1 jar or can organic black olives**
- **1 jar or can organic green olives**
- **Gluten-free flour**
- **Honey (local, of course)**
- **1 bottle prepared mustard (organic)**
- **Olive oil**
- **Apple cider vinegar**
- **Salt (see definitions)**
- **Pepper**
- **Coconut aminos**

Keep in mind that organic, pastured chicken is

expensive and worth every penny. This will be the most expensive item on your list for week one. Just know that two whole chickens are going to stretch into many meals. When I make this menu for my family of three people, the cost is $3.00 per person, per meal (not including pantry items). That's a phenomenal price for local, organic, "knowing my farmer," easy meals. Take that, fast food restaurants.

MEAL 1

Simple Roast Chicken

Preheat oven to 375°

2 whole chickens
1-2 Tbsp of lemon juice or 1 lemon quartered
1 cup water
1 cup chicken stock
1 cup white wine (optional)
Salt and pepper to taste

Rinse and pat the chickens dry. Remove neck and organ pack out of both chickens and save for another purpose. Place chickens side by side on a baking rack in a metal or a glass pan. Place the chickens breast side up, slather with olive oil and sprinkle with salt and pepper. Inside the cavity of each of the chickens, add one to two tablespoons of lemon juice or one lemon quartered, and two gloves of garlic smashed and diced. Place the chicken on a rack in a roasting pan. Fill the pan with your water, chicken stock and white wine.

Roast the chicken uncovered for 2 hours on the middle rack of the oven at 375 degrees. Remove from oven after two hours and let the chicken rest for 10 minutes. Eat roast chicken for dinner that night. Afterward, take the carcass of both chickens, strip any remaining meat off, and store these in 1 cup portions in resealable containers for meals later in the week.

After dinner and stripping the chickens of their meat, immediately place the remaining carcasses into the crock pot and then follow the Chicken Bone Broth Recipe on page 65. For two chickens, sometimes I have to do one batch of bone broth with one carcass, and then a few days later, remove the other chicken carcass from the refrigerator and use that for a 2nd batch of bone broth. This will depend on how big your crock pot is. No need to buy one, just adjust according to what you already have at your house.

Make sure you freeze half of your bone broth for recipes in the last part of the month.

Simple Baked Potatoes

1 potato per person
Olive oil to drizzle
Coarse Celtic salt

In the same oven as your roasting chicken, you will

bake your potatoes. You can add these during the last hour of cooking your chicken. Take one potato per person and wash it well. Slather it with olive oil and coarse salt and place it directly on the top rack of the oven (not in a pan). The drippings will fall into your chicken pan. Roast potatoes for one to one and a half hours. They will be crispy on the outside and soft on the inside. Eat with lots of pastured butter.

Zucchini and Yellow Squash Hash

2 cups peeled diced organic zucchini (or 2 small)
2 cups peeled diced organic yellow squash (2 small or 1 large)
1 tablespoon organic dill
3 tablespoons butter

Peel and slice both your zucchini and your yellow squash. Cut these rounds in half again. In a hot, cast-iron pan, melt three tablespoons of butter.
Salt and pepper generously. Fry your yellow squash and zucchini in the hot butter, scraping with a spatula and turning often. Add one tablespoon of dill in the last couple of minutes. Let it brown until the butter is gone and the zucchini/squash is almost crispy. Serve hot.

MEAL 2

CHICKEN AND WALNUT GREEN SALAD WITH CHERRIES AND HONEY MUSTARD DRESSING

Salad

1-2 heads romaine lettuce (washed and chopped finely)
1 cup shredded chicken (from Meal 1)
½ cup dried cherries (unsweetened)
2 oz organic goat cherries (unsweeted)
¼ cup organic walnuts (made into Crispy Nuts– see recipe on page 151)

Combine all ingredients together, top with the following dressing.

Honey Mustard Dressing

1 tablespoon organic mustard (dijon or regular)
1 tablespoon honey
¾ teaspoon salt
½ teaspoon black pepper
½ cup extra virgin olive oil

Add all ingredients into a mason jar, cover them with a lid, and vigorously shake until blended (it takes about one minute until the honey is incorporated). Drizzle it over the salad; toss it into a bowl with your other ingredients.

MEAL 3
BACON AND EGGS

If you haven't embraced bacon and eggs for dinner, you are in for a treat. This is an easy and fast meal.

Oven Bacon

1 package of good quality organic bacon (know your farmer, if possible.)
foil-lined cookie sheet

Cut the bacon in half and place on the foil. I make a little boat with the foil so the edges come up and hold all of the bacon grease.

Bake at 400 degrees for eighteen to twenty-two minutes. Remove and place the bacon on a paper towel to absorb any excess grease.

The bacon grease needs to be saved.. My mom and grandma always saved bacon grease, but not for the same reason that I do. I keep it for the health benefits of cooking with lard. Lard that comes from a pastured pig (see definitions) has as much Omega 3 fatty acid as salmon.

Take your foil boat and pour carefully into a glass jar while it is still liquid. After allowing it to cool, put a lid on your jar, and store it in the fridge.

Bacon is a favorite road trip food for my family. I will cook up a package of bacon, wrap in clean foil, and seal it in my airtight freezer bags. Unlike we've been told for years, bacon has been shown to be really good for you, providing excellent fats, proteins, and choline. There is even a company in the U.K. that has developed a car that runs on bacon grease. I use my Road King Cooker to heat up our bacon in the car. There's something decadent about eating hot bacon while on a long road trip. You can read more about snacking and eating on the go in my next book. Go to my online store to see Road King Cookers.

Eggs

1-2 eggs per person
1 tablespoon lard
¼ cup milk
salt and pepper to taste

Scrambled or over easy—you get to pick. Use local eggs from a great farmer. These chickens need to be out on pasture eating bugs and doing what chickens do (which is peck and scratch, eat and lay eggs.). Almost all chickens do eat some grains to keep them healthy, and to get enough protein, although, if forced, they will get all of their nutrients from grass and pasture if they have enough space. If your farmer does use some chicken feed, please ensure that your farmer uses organic/non-GMO/no-soy chicken feed. Please refer to Chapter 1 to read about the dangers of soy in eggs. .

Egg yolks from these special eggs are one of the healthiest foods on the planet. Embrace great eggs as a true healing food. Don't bother eating store-bought eggs—even the "good" organic kind. It's easy to find a local producer in every part of the country. If you need help, contact your local Weston A. Price chapter leader. The organization has lists of farmers they pass them along to you for free.

My husband went out to breakfast with his friend recently. He had a terrible time choking down the scrambled eggs from the restaurant where they were eating. Sadly, once you've been spoiled by real eggs (and real milk and real meat.), you can't go back to what most folks consider tasty.

Fruit and Sweeteners

Choose low-glycemic fruits when possible to keep your blood sugar stable. Once in a while, you can "treat" yourself to the sweeter fruits: pineapple, kiwi, mango, and banana. For the most part, though, stick with organic berries: blueberries, strawberries, raspberries, and blackberries. If you'd like, you can add diced green apple to the mix, which is also low on the glycemic index. The glycemic index measures the natural sugar content in foods.

Maintain healthy blood sugars to stay healthy. You want to keep your insulin from spikes and dips. Avoid processed sugar of all kinds, and use sweeteners (such as honey or maple syrup) in moderation. My "go to" sweeteners right now are coconut sugar and stevia. All stevia brands are not created equal. Some are highly processed and bleached, and some just taste awful. We use stevia Clear drops (non-flavored).

Studies are suggesting that mood regulation is related to steady blood sugar. Alzheimer 's disease in particular, is related to blood sugar regulation. Of course, we see in the media that Type 2 diabetes is an epidemic in modern America. Dialysis centers seem to be on every corner. Certain sugars, including high fructose corn syrup and/or white processed sugar, damage your gut lining. Keep that blood sugar steady to achieve real mental and physical health (Bland, 2014).

Maple syrup, honey, and coconut sugar are all much safer sweeteners because they are mostly sucrose sugar instead of fructose sugar. The body metabolizes sucrose much better than fructose. But do keep in mind that sugar is sugar and you should limit it as much as possible in your diet (Weil, 2016)

MEAL 4

Chicken and Brown Rice

1-2 cups brown rice (amount will be determined by the size of your family)
Use your Chicken bone broth from Meal 1 as your cooking liquid following rice package instructions
½ cup chopped organic carrots
½ cup organic peas
½ cup washed diced organic celery
OR
You can use any veggies (fresh or frozen) you prefer using the above amounts
½ teaspoon salt
¼ teaspoon black pepper
2 tablespoons butter

Before you go to bed the night before, you'll want to soak your rice in salt water. Rice, like any grain, has anti-nutrients in the outer grain that makes it difficult to digest. This is the part of the plant that protects it from insects. We can help to remove this phytic acid by soaking our grains overnight. Ancient peoples knew this and always prepared grains in a similar way.

To soak, add two cups of filtered water to one

teaspoon of salt in a pan and then add one to two cups of brown rice. Let the rice sit, covered, on the stove top until the next day when you are ready to use it. Rinse the rice very well before cooking.

Cook one to two cups of your brown rice in your chicken broth from Day 1, following package directions and depending on how many you are trying to feed. After forty minutes, when your rice is almost done, melt two tablespoons of butter in a separate skillet. Add chopped carrots, chopped celery, chopped peas (or any veggies of your choice) to the skillet. Steam until translucent.

Now, chop one cup of leftover roasted chicken that you cooked earlier in the week. In the last five minutes of your rice cooking, add your sautéed vegetables and your cooked chicken. Allow your rice to steam for five minutes with your veggies and chicken. Salt and pepper to taste.

Sweet Mustard Green Beans

1 pound organic green beans (fresh or frozen)
¼ teaspoon salt
2 tablespoons butter
2 tablespoons raw honey

In a small pot, boil two cups of filtered water and one-fourth of a teaspoon of good salt. Add rinsed green beans (I like fresh, and always organic—but make sure you pick off any stems). Cover with a lid and let boil for eight minutes. Remove from heat and drain. Add two tablespoons of good grass-fed butter. Mix in two tablespoons of raw honey (local, of course.) and two tablespoons of mustard. Stir until the ingredients are melted and incorporated. Eat immediately.

"Disease is the warning, and therefore the friend- not the enemy- of mankind."

-Dr. George S. Weger

MEAL 5

Smoky Red Lentil Soup

1 cup cooked chicken from Day 1 (chopped)
1 half gallon healing bone broth (made previously)
¾-1 cup red lentils (rinsed)
2 teaspoons smoked paprika
3-4 carrots (peeled and diced)
1-3 celery stalks (diced)
4 tablespoons butter
1 clove garlic (diced)
3-4 tablespoons onion (diced)
½ teaspoon salt

In a soup pot, melt butter on medium high heat. Add diced celery, diced carrots, garlic, and onion. Allow it to sauté until vegetables are somewhat transparent. Add broth, lentils, paprika and a half a teaspoon of salt. Cook on medium high with the lid on, for twenty minutes. Add additional salt and pepper to taste (I like mine salty).

Italian Salad

1 jar artichokes
1 jar green olives
1 jar black olives

1 tablespoon Italian dressing mix (see "Extras" section at the end of the book)
½ cup olive oil
¼ cup apple cider vinegar
1 tablespoon filtered water
4 ounces goat cheese or chevre (left over from Day 2 that you didn't use for the green salad)

In a glass quart jar, add drained olives, artichokes, and ingredients to make Italian salad dressing. Mix it all together and shake. Crumble the chevre and add it to the mixture. Allow flavors to mingle while your lentil soup is cooking.

MEAL 6

CHICKEN TERIYAKI STIR FRY

Sauce

4 tablespoons coconut aminos
2 tablespoons honey
2 Tablespoons grainy mustard

In a small bowl, mix your mustard, your coconut aminos, and your honey. Set aside.

Chicken Teriyaki

1 orange bell pepper (washed and chopped)
½ cup cooked broccoli
2 carrots (washed and chopped)

Heat a ten-inch, cast-iron skillet on medium high. Add one to two tablespoons of lard. Melt the lard and then add bell pepper and carrots. After these have "softened," add cooked broccoli, and one cup of cooked chicken from Day 1 (chopped or shredded).

Pour the sauce into your cast-iron skillet and heat through, allowing it to simmer for ten minutes.

Serve by itself, or over rice. This is awesome and fast.

MEAL 7

Chicken and Dumplings (One Pot Meal)

4 cups chicken bone broth
1 cup hot water
2½ cups cooked chicken
1 teaspoon salt
1 teaspoon Italian seasoning
1 teaspoon black pepper
½ teaspoon paprika
5 small potatoes (diced)
3 medium carrots (diced)
1 medium onion (diced)
1 tablespoon garlic (minced)
2 tablespoons butter

Sauté the celery, carrots, onion, and spices in a soup pot in two tablespoons of butter until slightly translucent. Add bone broth, hot water, and potatoes. Reduce to a simmer for ten to fifteen minutes or until your potatoes are cooked through

In a separate bowl, prepare your dumplings mixture.

Dumplings

1 cup gluten-free flour
1½ teaspoons baking powder
1½ teaspoons salt
1/4 teaspoon black pepper
1 tablespoon dried or fresh diced parsley
1 cup milk (or coconut milk)

Combine all ingredients and drop the dumpling mix by spoonfuls on top of the hot soup mix. Simmer the pot gently, uncovered for ten minutes. Then cover with a tight-fitting lid and simmer for fourteen more minutes.

MY STORY

Bread got me into this mess. Yes, I love bread. Often, we'd buy a loaf of hot French bread at our local grocery store and devour it on the way home. I love bread in almost every form and diligently ate it every day for the first thirty years of my life.

When my husband was suffering from the side effects of a brain injury he sustained in the Iraq war, he and I were together alone at the Wounded Warrior Clinic, and in and out of the hospital for two weeks. Being alone, for us, was a rare occurrence. There were no outside influences. Our child was with his grandparents, so we didn't have any other distractions. As my husband recovered, we spent lots of time at the hospital, waiting. My husband had no choice but to observe my mental state throughout the day, which allowed him to have an epiphany that would drastically affect my recovery.

In those days, I would wake up in the morning and be mentally and emotionally calm. This was normal for me. But as the day progressed, my mental state would worsen until about mid-afternoon when I was a terrified ball of mess. Anxiety would freeze me in my tracks and I would be fearful of the most ridiculous things. One of my fears was public restrooms and loud noises.

At the time, I was practicing the 80/20 rule. I ate 80 percent healthy (probably more like 50 percent, but in my mind I could still eat the yummy processed food I was addicted to and justify it). One day, my husband watched as I consumed a muffin at a coffee bar; then later the same day as I ate chicken nuggets from a fast food restaurant. My husband says I went from being calm and clear-headed to non-functioning in a matter of hours. Anxiety attacks, and a burning sensation in my brain literally melted me into a pile of sobs that afternoon after I ate these foods.

"What is happening to me?" I cried out. Frustrated, but clueless, I suffered through that day, as I had been doing for years by this point.

My husband turned toward me and said, "Every time you eat wheat, your brain crashes."

Of course, I didn't want to admit this. So, I tried a few experiments in the following days and sure enough, it was the wheat. In fact, it was probably a combination of wheat and the processed ingredients in what I was eating.

I stopped eating wheat that day and haven't eaten it since. I was tested for celiac disease, but don't have that condition. (Celiac is when a person is allergic to the protein found in wheat, and it is a serious condition. What's the difference between celiac disease and wheat intolerance? Celiac is an inability to digest the proteins in wheat and is, at its root, an autoimmune illness, meaning that the body's immune system is attacking the body. Celiac comes with a number of side effects, and is said to be a genetic condition.)

In my case, I have a wheat intolerance, which I've come to learn many people struggle with. We went to an event this past weekend and half of the children attending were gluten intolerant. I am not alone in not being able to properly digest wheat.

Personally, I didn't really believe wheat was so powerful (even knowing my own experience) in mood disorders until I became a neurofeedback specialist. I guess I needed to learn this lesson a couple of times. A neurofeedback specialist is a practitioner who assists people with brain issues of focus, memory, self-control, anxiety, and depression. After hearing about my own personal struggles, you can see why I was drawn to this therapy. Neurofeedback was phenomenal in helping me to cope with my symptoms. It's a tool that retrains the brain and it encourages the brain's neural pathways to function in a more optimal way. This therapy helped me greatly for two years in my journey to improve my health search.

When I saw the spectacular results it was achieving, I wanted to learn this way of healing and offer it to others. I went through a year-long internship, attended trainings, and worked with a wonderful doctor who shared his knowledge with me. After another year, he decided to retire and left me to run the clinic for him.

Several of my clients were children who had severe anger issues. They would throw chairs, become extremely aggressive with their siblings and parents, and exhibit episodes of extreme rage. When their health histories were examined or they were tested, these children would consistently show up with a wheat allergy. When wheat was eliminated, the behavior would disappear.

My son's wheat allergy looks different. We've also experimented with him. His main symptom is eczema on his upper arms and face. Since we've eliminated wheat from our diets, if he happens to have a little, watch out. Against my better judgment, I agreed to let him eat a homemade roll at a homeschool co-op we attended. They looked delicious and I didn't want to deprive him. They were homemade for goodness sake. My son ate that roll, and then had one of the biggest temper tantrums of his life. He became enraged (in front of many people who knew him as a kind and well-mannered young man). I couldn't believe the attitude he was giving me and I was forced to remove him from the room. As I was lecturing him on his lack of good behavior and asking him what in the world was wrong with him, I realized that it was the wheat talking. He had very little control over what he was saying or how he was acting. That was the last time he ate wheat and we have lived happily ever after.

I've discovered along the way that grains don't always agree with me, either; even properly prepared and gluten-free grains. (A properly prepared grain is a grain that is soaked overnight to eliminate the element in grain that makes it difficult to digest.) Limiting grains in my diet is what works best for me. Listen to your body. If you have an already compromised gut like I do, grains may be very difficult for you to eat.

There is an increasing body of evidence that supports grains causing inflammation throughout the body and in the brain (Perlmutter,2013). As a true Weston A. Price follower, I think grains are fine in moderation in a healthy body, and if they are properly prepared. Please see the many recipes on more ways to properly prepare your grains. My recipes can be adapted with an alternate side dish or you can eliminate certain portions of the recipes if you yourself are avoiding grains. The key here is –***listen to your own body***. You are in control and know what works best for you. Who knows? In a few years, I might decide that I need to avoid all grains, gluten-free or not.

For more information on soaking grains and properly preparing them, please see the Weston A. Price website at www.westonaprice.org.

CHAPTER 7:

Week Two:

Beef, It's What's On the Menu

Meal 1: Roast (bone-in recommended) with organic veggies

Meal 2: Barbeque beef with lemon broccoli

Meal 3: Taco Salad (this one doesn't need any extras.)

Meal 4: Waffles and sausage

Meal 5: Beef stew with rolls

Meal 6: Pot of beans

Meal 7: Hamburgers, fried apples, and baked cauliflower

GROCERY LIST FOR WEEK TWO

If you already have the items in your cupboard, then you're golden. Please just purchase the items that you need, which usually includes your meats and vegetables. Here we go.

- **1 bone-in, organic, pastured beef roast (approximately 3 pounds); Expensive but worth it.. You're going to get lots of meals out of this one item.**

- **2-3 pounds ground beef**
- **1 pound dried pinto beans (organic) or 32 ounces canned organic pinto beans**
- **Organic carrots**
- **Organic celery**
- **Organic broccoli**
- **Organic (a very small head)**
- **4 organic apples of any variety (Granny Smith preferred or a cooking apple)**
- **1 small onion (or dried onion flakes)**
- **2 organic tomatoes**
- **Organic canned garbanzo beans (8 ounces)**
- **Organic caned kidney beans (8 ounces)**
- **Raw cheddar cheese**
- ****optional: canned black olives**
- **1 package organic corn tortillas**
- **Sprouted spelt flour (One brand is a great product), or 1 package of gluten-free flour, or almond flour**
- **Red wine (your preference)**
- **Raw cheddar cheese**
- **Guacamole, or the ingredients to make guacamole**
- **Coconut oil**
- **Baking powder**
- **Honey**
- **Unsweetened ketchup**
- **Assorted spices**
- **Olive oil**
- **Butter**

FOR WEEK 2, COOK ONE OF THE FOLLOWING

Mama's Sprouted Spelt Bread

(Makes 1 large loaf)

3 cups organic sprouted spelt flour (you can sprout your own or buy a good brand like One)
2 cups organic whole buttermilk (make your own by adding 1 Tbsp of lemon juice to 2 cups of milk)
3 eggs
1 teaspoon salt
1/3 cup raw honey
2 teaspoons baking powder
¼ cup organic butter (melted)

Mix dry ingredients in one bowl. In another bowl, mix wet ingredients. Slowly add your wet ingredients into your dry ingredients a little at a time. Spread your batter into a buttered and floured loaf pan. Bake at 350 degrees for one and a half hours until a toothpick comes out clean. Serve with butter on top.

Or the no-grain option . . .

Almond Meal Biscuits

2½ cups almond flour (from soaked almonds using the "Crispy Nuts" recipe in the "Extras" section)

¾ teaspoon sea salt
¾ teaspoon baking soda
2 eggs
1/3 cup coconut oil (melted)
optional: add ½ teaspoon dried dill

Combine dry ingredients in a bowl. Combine wet ingredients in a separate bowl. Mix together without over-mixing. Using two tablespoons of batter, form into balls that are about two inches around. Press flat as needed. Place each on a Silpat-covered or parchment-lined cookie sheet. Bake for twelve to seventeen minutes until tops look slightly browned.

Let cool for thirty minutes and store in the refrigerator until needed and then warm when ready.

A note about cast-iron skillets: The best place to buy your cast-iron skillet is at an antique store, a garage sale, or from someone who refurbishes them. You can find lots of information online about restoring an old cast-iron skillet if necessary. They cost a little bit of money. My favorite size is a ten-inch skillet that I bought from a shop that restores old cast-iron. It's a Wagner brand, which I love. The reason I search for Wagner skillets is beacuse my first cast-iron skillet came from my Grandmother Distel. I scrub it out with a special green scrubbie and put it back on the hot stove top to dry. I never use soap of any kind. I often "season" my skillet with just a little lard or coconut oil to keep it non-stick. If you are suffering from anemia, a cast-iron skillet gives back by providing you with iron. I only use two frying pans now: my two cast-iron skillets.

I invested heavily in ceramic skillets a few years ago, but never use them now. The cast-iron is easy to clean without as much elbow grease and is just the right size for what I'm cooking. I love the flavor and how hot the skillet gets. We don't even put them away; they just live on the stovetop, clean and ready for the next meal.

Gluten Free Flours: There is a wide variety of gluten free flour on the market. The goal is to find a soaked and sprouted flour (because this removes the anti-nutrients of any grain, gluten containing or not).

Because gluten allergies are so common in this time in history, gluten free flours are readily available at any grocery store or health food store. My favorite have become brwon rice flour and my own combination of millet and sorghum. Although I love almond flour, it doesn't love me and so I need to eat it in moderation. I have found that rotating my non-gluten grains also helps. A wonderful local gluten free company taught me about combining millet and sorghum.

I don't necessarily like the modern gluten free flour blends. So any of them seem to resemble "processed food." My preference is to buy my flour from the "bulk" section of my health food store. Sally Fallon teaches us to "soak" our grains by adding our liquid to a recipe and some kind of acid like a teaspoon of lemon juice or apple cider vinegar and letting our batter sit over-night. This process helps us to easily remove anti-nutrients in our baked goods. I don't notice any taste difference due to adding the lemon juice. You do end up with a very nice textured baked good, though. It is only a personal prefer-ence, but I don't use much coconut flour in my own reci-pes.

MEAL 1

Bone In Pot Roast

1 bone-in roast
2 tablespoons lard
salt and pepper to taste

In a cast-iron skillet, melt two tablespoons of lard into a hot pan on medium-high heat. Sprinkle each side generously with salt and pepper. Brown each side of the roast for three to four minutes until a nice crust appears. Place browned roast in a Crock-Pot filled with the follow-ing:

2 teaspoons salt
1 teaspoon black pepper
6 cups filtered water

Cook on low for six to eight hours until the meat falls off the bone. Serve with baked potatoes, roasted vegetables, and a side of quinoa. Serve with rolls or bread you made for the week.

Brown your beef bone and place it immediately in your Crock-Pot for beef bone broth. Follow the directions and recipe in Chapter 5: Healing Broth #2 – Beef Bone Broth. Store in the refrigerator, removing fat after your broth has cooled. Use your beef broth recipes throughout the week and freeze any extra for another day.

A bone-in roast will cost you around $25.00 (or more) for a great pastured beef. It's worth it. I love tri-tip, or a lean chuck roast. If you can't get a bone-in roast, purchase your roast and a few beef bones. Even if you cook all the meals in this menu, you should still have plenty left to freeze in small portions and/or re-heat later for lunches. I freeze mine in one-cup portions because this amount works for my family of three. Adjust accordingly to the number you are feeding.

Buy a bone-in roast from a local rancher. I have to say, I'm spoiled in this category. Growing up, my grandparents owned a farm and cattle ranch. We always had beef and it was good quality beef. The first time I cooked hamburger from store-bought meat (which wasn't until I was in college), I thought it was just awful. Lucky for me, we always had good beef in the house when I visited home.

Now, many moons later, I have found an even more amazing tasting beef than what I grew up eating. My rancher is obsessed with the pasture where he grazes his cows. This obsession leads to an absolutely stellar cut of meat. I never knew beef could taste so incredible. My rancher sends long, descriptive, detailed emails about the state of his fields, what he's seeing grow in the pasture, and many names of grass that I've never heard of—names like "little blue-stem," "switch grass," and "Indian grass." I marvel at this Rancher who cares so much about my health and provides an amazing product.

Get out your Crock-Pot for this one. Brown your roast with a little butter in your cast-iron skillet. Turn it so that each side gets just a little brown. Salt and pepper generously. Then place in a Crock-Pot filled with water and ¼ cup of vinegar. Let the roast rest in cool water in the Crock-Pot with the ¼ cup of vinegar for thirty minutes which starts the process of pulling all the great minerals out of those bones. Cook on high for 4-6 hours. Your roast is done. Strip the meat off of the bones and return the bones to the broth mixture and cook for 2-3 additional days to make your healing bone broth. Eat the roast immediately for dinner.

MEAL 2

Easy BBQ Beef

4 cups shredded roast beef (left over from Day 1)

Sauce

In saucepan on low heat add:

1 cup unsweetened ketchup
½ sliced onion
2 teaspoons salt
1 tablespoon vinegar
1 tablespoon Worcestershire sauce
½ cup water
1 tablespoon raw honey
2 teaspoons chili powder
½ teaspoon black pepper

Simmer for fifteen minutes. Add roast to coat and heat through. Serve it by itself over Mama's Sprouted Spelt Bread (recipe on page 99) for an open face barbeque beef sandwich, or over Almond Meal Biscuits. This was my Mom's recipe and I ate it growing up. I've learned to take some of my favorite recipes and "health" them up. It's fairly easy to do and is definitely my "comfort food."

Lemon Broccoli

2 small heads organic broccoli or broccolini
2 cups filtered water
½ teaspoon salt
½ cup lemon juice
2 tablespoons butter
¼ teaspoon black pepper

Dice two large heads of raw broccoli into small pieces. Rinse well.

In a small pot, bring the two cups of filtered water and half a teaspoon of salt to a boil. Add washed and chopped broccoli florets and cook with a tightly covered lid for eight minutes. Remove from the heat and drain promptly.

Add butter and lemon juice, and additional salt and pepper. Optional: you can add one-fourth of a cup of sunflower seeds for crunch at the very end if you like.

MEAL 3

Home-Made Taco Seasoning Spice Mix

2 tablespoons chili powder (ancho chili powder from the Mexican grocery store is my favorite)
½ teaspoon garlic powder
½ teaspoon onion powder
½ teaspoon oregano
1 teaspoon paprika
1 tablespoon cumin
2½ teaspoons good salt

2 teaspoons black pepper

Mix all spices together. When you have browned one pound of ground beef in a skillet, add half a cup of water and two tablespoons of your mix. Stir and let simmer until the liquid is absorbed.

Mix a big batch of taco seasoning mix by quadrupling the recipe and then you can store it to be used in the future. Store it in a cool dry place in a glass jar.

Taco Salad

1 pound ground beef
½ teaspoon salt
¼ teaspoon pepper
1 tablespoon lard or butter
2 tablespoons of home-made taco seasoning spice mix (recipe on the previous page)
½ cup filtered water

In a hot skillet, add lard or butter until melted. Then brown one pound of ground beef. Stir as needed until the hamburger is thoroughly cooked through. Now add half a cup of water, and two tablespoons of your taco seasoning mix. Stir and lower your stove temperature until your mixture is at a simmer. Let it simmer for ten minutes, until the water has absorbed and cooked down. Add beans after they have been drained and rinsed.

Healthy fats are the key to a healthy mind and body. We need high levels of fat for every cell in our body. Most importantly, that fat plays a vital role in good brain health.

Your healthy fats for cooking are: cold-pressed coconut oil, extra virgin olive oil, lard from pastured bacon, tallow from grass-fed beef, and high quality butter from grass-fed cows (raw butter is best, but hard to obtain). Nut oils, sesame oil, and the like, are good fats, but very expensive, so they are not practical for use in everyday cooking.

- *Do not fry in extra virgin olive oil. The high heat destroys its good properties.*
- *Saturated fats, in spite of their bad rap, are actually good for you*
- *Avoid all other fats, especially trans fats.*
- *Eating healthy fats throughout the day helps to balance blood sugar.*

Home-Made Corn Chips

5 organic corn tortillas
2 cups coconut oil
sea salt

With a pizza cutter, divide it into eight to ten small pie-shaped wedges. Heat your cast-iron skillet with two inches deep of coconut oil. Allow it to get hot on medium-high heat. Gently drop the corn tortillas into the coconut oil. Flip in one minute. Remove to a paper towel and sprinkle with good Celtic sea salt. Store in an airtight container.

Why not use corn chips from the store, you ask? I haven't been able to find a brand that uses good fat. Good fats include butter, lard, olive oil, and coconut oil. This is changing, so hopefully someday soon that option will be available.

Building Your Taco Salad

½ cup guacamole (home-made or store-bought)
3 cups shredded lettuce
2 tomatoes (rinsed and diced)
Optional: 1 can black olives (drained)
1 can garbanzo beans
1 can black beans

Rinse and warm your garbanzo beans and black beans by adding them to your ground beef skillet after you have thoroughly cooked the hamburger. Place the lettuce, tomato, and olives into a bowl and toss. Add your seasoned ground beef and bean mixture on top and serve with a dollop of guacamole. This is a very filling dish.

MEAL 3

Easiest Beef Stew

1 cup cooked brown rice (soaked overnight and rinsed, previous to cooking)
8 carrots (chopped)
5 celery stalks (chopped)
3 yellow potatoes (peeled and cubed)
2 cloves of garlic
1 small onion (diced finely)
¼ stick butter (3 tablespoons)
8 cups beef broth
-½ cup red wine

In a stockpot, melt butter. Add onions, garlic, and veggies (except potatoes). Sauté until slightly translucent. Add beef stock (bone broth), potatoes, and rice at this time. Let it simmer for twenty minutes. Add two to three cups of chopped or shredded roast beef that was left over from Meal 1. Serve hot.

MEAL 4
WAFFLES

Use "Dorothy's Famous Pancake Recipe" below. This recipe works for both pancakes and waffles, with no changes.

Dorothy's Famous Pancakes

This is my mom's recipe and I don't know how we'd get by in our house without it.

2 cups brown rice flour, or sprouted flour (spelt, wheat, buckwheat—your family's preference), or Bob's Red Mill Gluten-Free Blend
3 teaspoons baking powder
2 pastured eggs
2 cups of raw milk
¼ cup of coconut oil (melted)

In a bowl, combine baking powder and eggs with a spoon. Stir thoroughly and let foam for two minutes. Add flour and milk. Get your skillet hot, on medium-high heat, and add coconut oil to your skillet. Allow it to melt and then pour that into your batter. Stir until well-mixed, but try not to over-mix the batter. This is a great batter to prepare overnight, add 1 teaspoon of lemon juice, and let the anti-nutrients in grain break down in the fridge. You can easily cook up the pancakes in the morning.

Add by a quarter of a cup at a time into your skillet. When the edges look slightly dry, flip. I make a big batch each week and store it in the fridge. These are snacks, "bread" at dinner time, and breakfast treats. Just warm them up and let your imagination go.

The ways my family likes to eat either pancakes or waffles:
-good butter and real maple syrup
-almond butter and a sliced banana
-a big dollop of real butter with apple butter on top

These pancakes are road trip favorites, too. I make up a batch, and then freeze them in my air-sealed bags. Place a piece of waxed paper between each. Use the re-sealable bags in which you can suck out the air. These are great in a hotel, warmed. We often stay at a hotel where they have some kind of breakfast (which I have no interest in). But usually they will have peanut butter and bananas. We use these on top of our home-made pancakes and that allows us to have a great breakfast while traveling.

And lastly, during a regular week, we keep Dorothy's pancakes made and in the fridge so we can pull them out and warm up a few when we just don't have time to cook. Then we add the things we like—a big dollop of butter, applesauce on mine, real maple syrup on my husband's and son's, and we have a delish breakfast.

You can add one-fourth a cup of fresh blueberries (washed) if you like, as the last ingredient to your batter and then cook in your skillet or waffle maker.

Home-Made Sausage Patties

1 pound ground beef (pastured)
1 teaspoon salt
¾ teaspoon black pepper
1 teaspoon sage
1 teaspoon thyme
¼ teaspoon rosemary
1 tablespoon coconut sugar
¼ teaspoon nutmeg
¼ teaspoon cayenne pepper

Combine ground beef with all the other ingredients and let it chill for one hour to mingle the flavors. Shape into two-inch patties and cook in a cast-iron skillet with one to two tablespoons of lard until it is browned and cooked through on all sides.

MEAL 5

Pot of Beans

1 pound pinto beans (dried) or 2 cans pinto beans (the larger size can)
1 teaspoon salt (or 2 teaspoons, in you prefer)
1 teaspoon baking soda
2 cups paleo ketchup (unsweetened or sweetened with coconut sugar)

Take dried pinto beans. Remove any debris or broken/misshapen beans and soak the rest in a bowl of filtered water (enough to cover beans by four inches—beans will absorb water and double in size overnight) with one teaspoon of salt and one teaspoon of baking soda. Let it sit overnight, for twelve hours. When you are ready to start cooking, rinse the beans thoroughly. They will no longer be spotted. Instead, they will be reddish in color. My sister-in-law says to rinse them until you don't see bubbles if you want to reduce flatulence.

In a large soup pot, generously cover the soaked beans with filtered water (four inches over the top of the beans). Let them simmer with two teaspoons of salt for one hour. Then test the beans to see if they are done. Keep simmering as needed until they are soft. Add two cups of paleo ketchup (or ketchup sweetened with coconut sugar). I purchase mine at our local paleo store—Evolve Paleo from Kansas City.

Serve with some of your yummy bread from earlier in the week with generous amounts of butter.

MEAL 6

Seasoned Hamburgers

This is my family's version of hamburgers. We love having a batch of these in the fridge to re-heat.
Here's my interpretation.

1 pound ground beef
2 teaspoons paprika
1¼ teaspoons salt
¼ teaspoon garlic powder
¼ teaspoon onion powder
¼ teaspoon love

Mix the thawed ground beef and all of the spices together. Form small patties with approximately a two-inch diameter. Fry them in a #10 cast-iron pan or any skillet on med or high heat, flipping them twice to cook evenly. I often brown the outsides very nicely, and then add one inch of filtered water to the bottom of my skillet and cover it with a tight-fitting lid. I find this steams the meat and cooks it all the way through.

A serving is three to four patties, ketchup, mustard, and diced pickles on top. Who needs a bun?

Fried Apples

This is a particular favorite of mine. It's like apple pie filling without the crust.

2-3 soft apples
3 tablespoons butter
cinnamon to sprinkle

Choose a softer apple variety, like Cameo. Wash, peel, and cut them into wedges. Fry them in your skillet in a generous amount of good butter on med to high heat. Stir as they brown until they are cooked through and have a nice "crust." Add a generous sprinkling of cinnamon in the last minute of cooking. This takes approximately ten minutes. Serve hot. . If you put these in the refrigerator and re-heat for later, it's just like eating apple pie filling. They get nice and soft.

Baked Cauliflower

1 head organic cauliflower washed and cut into florets
3 tablespoons olive oil
1 tablespoon dry ranch dressing mix (see recipe in "Extras" section in the back of the book)

In a bowl, mix olive oil and ranch dressing dry mix together with cauliflower. Place it on a lined baking sheet, (I use Silpat) and roast at 400 degrees for twenty to twenty-five minutes, or until the cauliflower is soft.

MEAL 7

SPAGHETTI WITH SPAGHETTI SQUASH "NOODLES"

Sauce

1 pound ground beef
2 tablespoons lard
¼ teaspoon salt
¼ teaspoon black pepper
1 jar of no sugar added organic spaghetti sauce

Brown one pound of ground beef or ground buffalo in a cast-iron skillet with two tablespoons of lard. Add one jar of good spaghetti sauce to the browned and seasoned meat.

This might be one of my most complicated recipes (I say this tongue in cheek). I buy a good brand of sauce (organic with no sugar added); that's it. Warm sauce and meat through and serve over squash.

Spaghetti Squash

1 organic spaghetti squash
3 tablespoons butter
salt and pepper to taste

Preheat your oven to 400 hundred degrees. Wash the spaghetti squash. Cut it in half and remove the seeds. In a glass baking dish, add two inches of filtered water to the bottom. Place the squash, cut side down, into the dish and bake at 400 hundred degrees for forty minutes. Allow it to cool slightly. Remove it from the pan and with two forks and "flake" the squash away from the skin. Scrape the squash into a bowl and then add three tablespoons of butter. Salt and pepper to taste. Discard the skin. Serve it smothered in the sauce recipe (above).

This meal goes great with a green salad.

The controversy with microwaves

- *A number of studies show that when you use your microwave, you kill the living nutrients.*
- *The November 2003 issue of The Journal of the Science of Food and Agriculture revealed that broccoli that had been cooked in the microwave showed a 97 percent reduction in its beneficial antioxidants. Steamed broccoli lost 11 percent of its antioxidants.*
- *A 1999 Scandinavian study found that microwaving asparagus spears caused a reduction in vitamin C.*
- *As little as sixty seconds of microwave heating was enough to inactivate alliinase, garlic's primary active ingredient against cancer.*
- *A Japanese study by Watanabe demonstrates that six minutes of microwave cooking killed thirty to forty per-*

cent of the B12 in milk.

Microwaves heat food by causing water molecules to resonate at very high frequencies. This then turns into steam to heat the food. While this can give you a hot cup of coffee in a matter of seconds, it also causes a change in the food's chemical structure. "Microwaving distorts and deforms the molecules of whatever food or other substance you subject to it. But even if there's nothing wrong with your microwave, keep in mind that standing a foot away from it while it's running can expose you to upwards of 400 milliGauss, and a mere 4 milliGauss has been firmly linked to leukemia."

If you do decide to microwave, keep in mind that you need to step away from it when its running. "Also, since your eyes are known to be particularly susceptible to microwave radiation (high microwave exposures are known to cause cataracts), I recommend stepping away from your microwave while it's in use." (Paraphrased, Mercola, 2012)

CHAPTER 8

Week 3: Here Fishy, Fishy

Meal 1: Clam Chowder with Fruit

Meal 2: Yellow Split Pea Soup with Cinnamon Stevia "Chips"

Meal 3: Maple Syrup Salmon with Steamed Broccoli

Meal 4: Tuna Salad and Fruit

Meal 5: Salmon over Green Salad

Meal 6: Salt and Pepper Pork Roast, Mashed Potatoes, and Green Peas

Meal 7: Puff Pancake with Apple and Blueberry Topping and Oven Bacon

Seafood is important because it has very high vitamin content. Clams and oysters contain the highest levels of B vitamins of any food. Of course, we've all heard of the benefits of Omega 3 fish oils. The level of nutrients is phenomenal. But, our oceans are polluted and the fish absorbs these toxins. Fortunately for you, I've found some great comanies and some fabulous recipes that will make adding seafood to your diet easy and affordable.

Seafood is mysterious to me. I know it is extremely beneficial, but I'm a landlubber. I grew up in the mountains in the middle of the country. Colorado just isn't known for its fresh seafood. Finding a good seafood supplier is challenging. You want wild seafood, from pure waters, and at a great price, too. Easy, right? I order my seafood like I do my beef. We belong to a bulk order club. I let everyone know I'm buying seafood and they all chime in with their orders. The more we buy, the more we save. Shipping is free for these large orders and I am supporting an ethical seafood company that I trust. See "Resources" on page 166 for wonderfully sourced seafood.

GROCERY LIST

- **Carrots**
- **Yellow potatoes**
- **Organic heavy cream**
- **9-10 fresh or frozen clams (from a great source please.)**
- **Jumbo prawns (9-12 or 3-4 per person is perfect)**
- **Brown rice**
- **2 salmon filets (or ½ per person)**
- **Maple syrup**
- **Garlic**
- **Broccoli**
- **Yellow split peas (go to the bulk bin.)**

- **Chicken stock (20 ounces) from your "Winner, Winner, Chicken Dinner" batch that you have in your freezer**
- **48 ounces canned pinto beans**
- **Canned tuna**
- **Canned salmon**
- **Olive oil**
- **Apple cider vinegar**
- **Italian dressing dry mix (see Recipe on page….)**
- **Blueberries**
- **2-3 apples**
- **Capers**
- **Lettuce (Romaine recommended)**
- **Pork tenderloin**
- **Celery**
- **Onion**
- **Brown rice tortillas**
- **Assorted spices**
- **Green peas**
- **Gluten-free flour**
- **Bacon**
- **1 small bunch chard**
- **1 small fennel**

MEAL 1
CLAM CHOWDER

Clam Chowder is full of kabam-packed nutrients. Clams contain some of the highest amounts of B-vitamin levels and Zinc you can get. I make a big batch of clam chowder every now and again and freeze it in individual, four-ounce containers I use stainless steel condiment cups from a big box store.

I heat one each day (not in the microwave, of course.) and that is my “multivitamin.” On the days when I am making my big batch of clam chowder individual servings, I serve clam chowder for dinner, too. I just love eating my vitamins, don’t you?

Clam Chowder Multivitamin Stew

8-10 clams (live or frozen)
4-5 yellow potatoes
1 quart of organic heavy whipping cream
4 tablespoons butter
3 stalks celery cleaned and diced
¼ cup diced onion
2 tablespoons minced garlic

Steam clams in boiling water for two to three minutes. Do not over boil. Remove them from the heat. When the shells pop open, remove them from the inside, reserving your clam liquid (the water you boiled them in). Dice the clams finely.

In a soup stock pan, melt the butter. Add onions, diced celery, garlic, and diced carrots until just translucent. Then add peeled and quartered potatoes. Simmer until the potatoes are soft, stirring them occasionally. Add clams and one-third of a cup of clam liquid at the very end, along with salt and pepper to taste.

Serve with rolls (see week 1) or a side of fruit.

MEAL 2

Yellow Split Pea Soup

2 cups cleaned and rinsed yellow split peas
20 ounces healing chicken broth
4 cups diced chard
1 diced fennel
½ teaspoon good salt
¼ teaspoon black pepper
4 tablespoons butter

After removing the debris from your lentils, soak them overnight. Melt the butter in large stock pot. Add cleaned and diced chard and fennel to the butter. Cook for two minutes and then add broth, rinsed split peas, salt, and pepper. Enjoy hot with cinnamon/stevia chips.

Cinnamon Stevia Chips

3-4 brown rice tortillas
1 tablespoon cinnamon
1 tablespoon stevia powder
1 cup coconut oil

With a pizza cutter, cut tortillas into small pie-shaped wedges (to resemble corn chips). In a large cast-iron skillet, melt one cup of coconut oil. When the oil is hot, add brown rice tortilla chips. Fry on each side for one to two minutes, flipping halfway through. Place them on a paper towel and sprinkle with cinnamon and then stevia powder. I keep a small container of the cinnamon/stevia mixture in my kitchen that is already mixed with one teaspoon of cinnamon to one teaspoon stevia.

"The human body heals itself and nutrition provides the resources to accomplish the task."

-Roger Williams Ph.D.

MEAL 3

Maple Syrup Salmon

¼ cup maple syrup
¼ cup Bragg's liquid aminos
1 tsp garlic powder *or* 2 cloves minced

Place one to two salmon filets in a resealable container with one-fourth of a cup of maple syrup, Bragg's liquid amino acids, and two cloves of minced garlic. Let it marinate for about two hours. Don't let it marinate too long. Unlike beef or chicken, salmon can't marinate for more than eight hours, otherwise you're turning it into sashimi (a kind of sushi). Two hours of marinating is plenty for our recipe.

Place salmon, skin side down, in a glass baking dish and put it in the oven at 400 degrees for twenty minutes. Serve hot with the Lemon Broccoli Recipe found on page 105.

MEAL 4

Tuna salad

1 can or pouch of sustainable tuna
3 pickles (diced)
mayonnaise (make your own or find a good source with good fats)
2 celery stalks (washed and diced)

Combine all ingredients above and mash them with a fork. Serve over greens, like red leaf lettuce. Eat with a side of fruit (grapes are my favorite).

MEAL 5

Salmon over Green Salad

2 pouches or cans smoked salmon
2 tablespoons capers
2 tablespoons olive oil
1 tablespoon dry dill
1 tablespoon lemon juice

Mix all ingredients and serve them over washed and diced greens, like romaine lettuce.

Serve with a side of ripe raspberries, washed and sprinkled with cinnamon.

MEAL 6

Salt and Pepper Pork Loin

1 pork loin (2-4 pounds)
2 teaspoons salt
1 teaspoon black pepper

My preference is to grill outside, but another option is to bake it in the oven. To bake, preheat oven to 325 degrees. In a hot skillet or cast-iron pan, with one to two tablespoons good lard, brown the sides of the pork roast. Place it in a shallow baking dish and bake for one and a half to two hours, or until your meat thermometer reads 155 degrees. On your outdoor grill, cook on medium high, rotating every eight minutes until your meat thermometer reads 155 degrees.

A note about meat thermometers; I don't have a lot of kitchen gadgets but I do have a digital meat thermometer. They are inexpensive and a fantastic kitchen tool to own.

Mashed Potatoes

4 yellow potatoes (organic)
½ teaspoon salt
3 tablespoons butter
¼-1/2 cup milk

Wash and peel the potatoes. In a pot, add salt and fill with filtered water about three-fourths of the way full. Bring it to a full boil. Cut potatoes into bite-size pieces, then drop them into a pot of boiling water. Let boil for fifteen minutes, until potatoes are soft (you should be able to put a fork in them). Drain the pot. Add butter and milk, then mash the potatoes with a masher. I like mine slightly less thick. The starch in the potatoes will thicken them up.

Serve with more butter and salt and pepper to taste.

Green Peas

frozen or fresh green peas (1/2 pound)
2 cups filtered water in a saucepan
½ teaspoon salt

Bring the water to a boil. Add peas and salt and place a lid on top. Reduce to medium/high allowing it to boil for eight minutes. Drain the water, add butter and serve immediately.

MEAL 7

Puff Pancake with Fruit Topping

4 tablespoons butter
4 tablespoons coconut sugar
½ teaspoon cinnamon
¾ cup whole milk
3 eggs
½ cup gluten free flour
½ teaspoon salt
½ teaspoon vanilla extract

Preheat the oven to 400 degrees. In a ten-inch cast-iron skillet, melt the butter and stir in one tablespoon of coconut sugar and cinnamon.

In a separate bowl, combine other the ingredients. Pour them into the cast-iron skillet and bake for fifteen to twenty minutes. It should be puffed and slightly browned on top when you take it out.

Fruit Topping

2 apples (washed, peeled, cored, and diced)
1 cup berries (washed); (blueberries, blackberries, raspberries, or strawberries)
2 tablespoons coconut oil

In a cast-iron skillet (I use my smaller six-inch cast-iron skillet for the topping), melt the coconut oil. Add berries and apples and fry until they become soft. Optional: add one-fourth of a cup of "crispy nuts" (this could be walnuts, almonds, or any variety you prefer). Serve the fruit topping on the puff pancake.

Oven Bacon

1 package of high quality bacon

Pre-heat the oven to 400 degrees. If you're doing the puff pancake, you can put the bacon in at the same time. Cut the bacon strips in half and place them on a foil-lined cookie sheet, allowing the foil to come up on the sides. Place in a single layer.

Bake it for twenty minutes until brown and crispy. Remove the bacon immediately from drippings and place it on a paper towel. With your foil boat, pour the bacon drippings (lard) into your lard jar and keep it refrigerated until you're ready to use it for another recipe.

CHAPTER 9

Week 4:
Mix it Up

Meal 1: Shish Kabobs

Meal 2: Omelets and Fruit

Meal 3: Bean Chowder, Almond Flour Biscuits

Meal 4: Chicken and Rice Stew, Small 3-Bean Salad

Meal 5: Spicy Hot Sausage and Potatoes, with Easy Baked Veggies

Meal 6: Miranda's Secret Recipe Chili, and Cast-Iron Skillet Cornbread

GROCERIES FOR THIS WEEK:

- **1 pound round steak**
- **½ pound hamburger**
- **Cherry tomatoes**
- **Pineapple**
- **Raw cheddar**
- **Organic corn grits**
- **Eggs (pastured organic)**
- **Assorted fruit**
- **Dried chili red chili**

- **Salt**
- **Pepper**
- **Dried parsley**
- **Dried garlic**
- **Pinto beans (I like canned, but you can use dried if you prefer)**
- **Almond flour**
- **Fresh dill**
- **2 cups frozen chicken (from previous "Winner, Winner, Chicken Dinner" week)**
- **16 ounces frozen chicken broth (from previous "Winner, Winner, Chicken Dinner" week)**
- **Potatoes**
- **Zucchini**
- **Squash**
- **Canned tomatoes**
- **Sprouted spelt**
- **Butter**
- **Baking powder (aluminum-free)**
- **Bamboo skewers**

Shish Kabobs

12 bamboo skewers
1 package organic grape or cherry tomatoes (they have fun colors like dark purple, yellow, orange, and red.)
1 cup organic teriyaki sauce
organic pineapple cut into 1-inch cubes

round steak cut into cubes (or you can use any cut of beef you prefer)
1-2 tablespoons lard or butter

Once you have your meat cut into cubes, marinate overnight in teriyaki sauce and place it in a sealable container overnight. Assemble your kabobs, alternating your marinated meat and veggie, meat and veggie.

Before cooking, heat your cast-iron skillet on medium. Add lard or butter and let it melt. Place the kabobs into your hot skillet and brown on each side for three to five minutes. Do a quarter turn with tongs until cooked through. Serve hot, over brown rice.

"All that man needs for health and healing has been provided by God in nature, the challenge of science is to find it."
-Philippus Theophrastus Bombast that of Aureolus Paracelsus (1493-1541)

Apples 'n Almonds

2 apples of your choice (Granny Smith or cooking apples preferred)
¼ cup crispy almonds (See "Extras" section for Crispy Nuts Recipe)
2 tablespoons honey

Wash the apples. With the skin left on, core, slice, and dice them. Add one-fourth of a cup of crispy almonds and two tablespoons of good local honey. Mix and let flavors merge for ten minutes.

Omelets

Omelets are easy to make and yummy. They also make a nice, fast meal.

2 eggs per omelets
3 tablespoons raw milk or cream
salt and pepper to taste
fresh dill
1 tablespoon raw gouda cheese (grated or chopped into small pieces—or you can choose the cheese you prefer)
1 tablespoon lard

In a bowl, add eggs, milk, fresh dill, and gouda cheese (chopped into little pieces or grated) Heat a cast-iron skillet on medium until hot. Melt one tablespoon of lard. Turn heat down to low and add the egg mixture. Cook for about three minutes and flip one half over the other half. Allow to cook for one to two minutes longer. Then flip the entire omelet and cook for an additional one to two minutes. Serve hot with a side of cantaloupe. My favorite for fast food.

You can do a number of variations to this recipe. Add whatever you like—onions, mushrooms, peppers, or even top it with hollandaise sauce. You can fry bacon, ham, or sausage and serve with it, too.

"According to the World Health Organization (WHO), America is the 37th healthiest nation in the world. Basically the American Medical Association's team is in 37th place. When was the last time you took the word of the 37th place team as Gospel?"

-Steve Plog, Founder,
Results Project

Bean Chowder

2 16-ounce cans pinto beans (organic)
1-2 teaspoons salt
½-1 teaspoon pepper
4 cups filtered water
1 tablespoon lard

In your pot, add all of your ingredients, rinsing your soaked beans especially well until there are no bubbles visible before you add these. Let your mixture simmer for twenty minutes. With a potato masher, mash your beans (smashed beans, I call them) while they are just a little hot.. Let it simmer for an additional five minutes. Add more salt and pepper as needed. Serve with organic sour cream and bacon crumbled on top.

"It seems that some consideration should be given to the cause of our mounting physical disabilities, but instead of going to the root of our troubles- wrong habits of eating and drinking- we rush to the medicine shelf and smother our uncomfortable and distressing symptoms under an avalanche of pills, potions and palliatives."

-Brother Roloff

Almond Flour Biscuits

2½ cups sprouted almond flour
¾ teaspoon sea salt
¾ teaspoon baking soda
1 cup raw cheese grated (parmesan or cheddar—you pick.)
1 tablespoon rosemary or dill
2 cloves garlic (minced) or 1 teaspoon dried garlic powder
2 tablespoons organic Dijon mustard
2 free-range eggs
1/3 cup of coconut oil (melted)

Preheat oven to 350 degrees. Use a Silpat cookie sheet liner or parchment paper. In a large bowl, combine dry ingredients. In a second bowl, whisk wet ingredients. Stir the wet ingredients slowly into the dry ingredients until they are thoroughly mixed. Form balls using two tablespoons. Flatten with a spoon and leave two inches between each to allow for expansion while baking. Bake twelve to seventeen minutes, until golden brown. Let cool for thirty minutes.

Variations can include adding cinnamon and two tablespoons of maple syrup, instead of the Dijon and the herbs. Then sprinkle with cinnamon after you have them flattened, but before baking or you can leave them plain and add an all-fruit jam and butter to make traditional biscuits.

Chicken and Rice Soup

24 ounces healing chicken stock (also known as bone broth—that you have frozen from a previous meal)
2 cups rice (cooked); I like brown Rice, soaked, rinsed, and cooked
4-5 carrots (diced)
4 stalks celery (diced)
potatoes, zucchini, yellow squash (peeled and diced)
2 teaspoons salt
½ teaspoon black pepper
3 tablespoons butter or 3 tablespoons lard
3 teaspoons garlic (minced)
¼ cup onions (red are mighty nice)
1-2 cups simple roasted chicken (frozen from a previous day)

In a stockpot, melt butter or lard. Add garlic, onion, and diced veggies. Sauté until somewhat translucent (two to five minutes). Pour in broth, rice, salt, and pepper, then cook for ten minutes at a simmer. Add roasted and shredded (or diced chicken) to the pot in the last few minutes (otherwise it will cook into tiny little pieces). Heat through and you're done. Easy peasy. Serve hot and enjoy.

Three-Bean Salad

1 8-ounce can green beans (organic)
1 8-ounce can garbanzo beans
1 8-ounce can kidney beans

Rinse your cans of beans well until you don't see any bubbles. Combine all of them in a bowl or glass jar and allow them to marinate in Italian salad dressing mix (see recipe in the "Extras" section) for at least twenty minutes.

Spicy Hot Sausage and Potatoes

3 yellow potatoes (also called Yukon gold)
2 tablespoons lard or butter
summer sausage (sliced and chopped); we like Organic Valley brand
½ cup organic salsa (we like Frontera Brand, mild)
¼ teaspoon salt
1/8 teaspoon black pepper
½ cup filtered water

Wash and slice potatoes into bite-size pieces. In a cast-iron skillet, add lard until it melts. Add potatoes into the skillet and salt and pepper. Pan fry potatoes until they are browned, then add sausage, water, and salsa. You can add canned beans of any kind-pinto or black beans are good choices- rinse well and add to the pan with all other ingredients. Stir. Reduce heat to simmer and cover with a tight-fitting lid. Allow it to simmer for ten to fifteen minutes. When you can pierce the potatoes with a fork, they are soft enough. Your dish is ready to eat.

"An apple a day keeps the doctor away."
-Your mother

Easy Baked Veggies

2 cups raw veggie (washed, diced) of your choice. You can use cauliflower florets, broccoli florets, green beans, potatoes, turnips—anything you like for this recipe.
1 tablespoon dry ranch dressing mix (see "Extras" section in the back of the book).

In a bowl, mix your vegetable of choice with one tablespoon of ranch dry mix (recipe in "Extras" section) and two tablespoons of good olive oil. Stir to coat and then place the entire mixture on a Silpat covered cookie sheet (or lined with parchment). Bake at 400 degrees for twenty to twenty-five minutes. Enjoy.

Miranda's Secret Recipe Chili

1 pound ground beef
2 tablespoons onion (minced) or minced dried onion
2 tablespoons chili powder
2 teaspoons salt
2 teaspoons oregano
1 16-ounce can stewed tomatoes
1 8-ounce can tomato juice or 1 pint canned tomato juice
2 cans organic kidney beans (drained and rinsed)
¼ cup apple cider vinegar

Brown ground beef in a cast-iron skillet on medium high. When the meat is cooked through (I like mine very browned), add to a soup pot with all other ingredients. Bring to a slow boil for fifteen minutes. Remove from heat and enjoy. This recipe is great to freeze or to double.

Cast-Iron Skillet Corn Bread

1½ cups cornmeal (organic and non-GMO)
½ cup all-purpose gluten-free flour
1 teaspoon salt
1 teaspoon baking powder
1 egg
4 tablespoons butter
1½ cups buttermilk
4 tablespoons honey

Pre-heat oven to 400 degrees.Mix all dry ingredients together in a mixing bowl. In a small saucepan, melt the butter, add milk, (and one teaspoon of lemon juice to make buttermilk), and four tablespoons of honey until the honey is just melted.

Add to dry mix. Mix thoroughly and place in a ten-inch cast-iron pan. Place pan in the oven for twenty to twenty-five minutes until the top is just browned. Allow to cool for five minutes. Serve with extra butter and honey on top.

SOME THINGS TO NOTE

I like to make a bigger batch each week than what we're planning to eat. If I can, I like to freeze these meals and store them for a day when we are under the weather, tired, or taking a trip and need something frozen. I am in a rhythm with what I cook. For some folks, eating beef for many days in one particular week isn't fun. If you prefer variety, that's fine. Instead, cook ahead and freeze the various weeks. Then you can mix and match beef with chicken, add in pork, or mix it up in any way you like.

I eat a fair amount of starches, which is a no-no on the "Gut and Psychology Syndrome Diet" (GAPS)—a therapy designed by Natasha Campbell-McBride. If you are using GAPS protocol, please adjust accordingly. You can adapt my entire meal plan to GAPS. This therapy is for intensive gut healing. If you'd like more information on GAPS, please visit www.gapsdiet.com.

"God, in His infinite wisdom, neglected nothing and if we would eat our food without trying to improve, change or refine it, thereby destroying its life-giving elements, it would meet all requirements of the body."

-Jethro Kloss

EXTRAS

Crispy Nuts

I've said it before, but nuts and grains have a coating on them that prevents digestion. In order to help your body break them down, you should always soak grains and nuts. Here's how you do it.

Soak four cups of nuts (any kind of nut) in filtered water with two tablespoons of salt (good salt, please, with color like Redmond's Salt). Allow them to soak overnight. Rinse them well in the morning and place them on a cookie sheet in a low-temperature oven (as low as your oven will go. My oven will go as low as 170 degrees). Allow them to remain in the oven four hours, or until dried out. Store in an airtight, glass container.

Italian Dressing Dry Mix

7½ teaspoons garlic powder
5 tablespoons onion powder
10 tablespoons dried oregano leaves
5 tablespoons dried parsley
10 tablespoons salt (like Redmond's Brand)
5 teaspoons black pepper
5 teaspoons dried basil leaves

1¼ teaspoons dried thyme leaves
2½ teaspoons dried celery flakes

Mix it all together and store in an airtight glass container (I use a one-quart canning jars). Use as needed for many recipes.

Italian Dressing

2 tablespoons of dry mix (above)
2 tablespoons water
½ cup of olive oil
¼ cup of good quality vinegar (like Bragg's or Mother's brand)

Place in a container with a lid (I use a pint jar) and shake vigorously. Serve immediately.

Ranch Dressing Dry Mix

15 tablespoons dried onions (minced)
7 teaspoons parsley flakes
4 teaspoons salt
1 teaspoon garlic powder

Mix it all together and store in a glass container until needed.

"Health requires healthy food."

-Roger Williams

Ranch Dressing

2 tablespoons dry mix (above)
1 cup mayonnaise
Make sure your mayonnaise has a healthy fat, like olive oil. Do not use a brand that uses canola oil, safflower oil, or soybean oil. Please see the section on healthy fats.
1 cup buttermilk

To make buttermilk, add one teaspoon of lemon juice to your milk.
Mix it all thoroughly and let it sit for fifteen minutes to combine flavors. Always use organic spices to create your mixes. Natural grocers in my area carry great bulk items or Frontier online.

"When you see the Golden Arches you are probably on the road to the Pearly Gates."

-William Castelli, MD - Director, Framingham Heart Study

MY STORY

I am the face of mental illness. If you asked me fifteen years ago if I had mental illness, I would have vehemently denied it. First of all, it's embarrassing. It seems like a weakness that I should be able to overcome if I only try hard enough. In the beginning, I was determined to "fix this" with positive thinking. I just knew I could do it in my own strength and I could overcome my irrational fears and thoughts. The fact is, when I ate processed food, I fell apart mentally and emotionally. I experienced extreme anger and I wanted to hurt people—for real.

I've learned that when I am feeling fearful, afraid

to drive, or develop an irrational fear, that this is simply a symptom of my entire system being off-balance. Yes, even I forget that I need nutrients when I'm travelling or out of my rhythm. I have to be reminded to go back and start at the beginning; sauerkraut, bone broth and kefir.

You will undoubtedly have different challenges than I have had. I am healed, but I am at risk for relapse if I don't guard my gut and the food I put into my body. I hope you come away from this book with hope that any type of mental illness has a root (and it isn't because you aren't strong enough, wise enough, or smart enough) of nutrient deficiency. It can be healed. Nutrients might not be the entire picture. Counselors are wonderful resources who are called to assist us on this journey. I couldn't have healed if I hadn't pursued emotional and spiritual healing, too.

When people ask me how they should heal, I advise them to pray about it. We are such unique creatures; each one of us as different as our fingerprints. God knows the next step you need to take, and if you yield to his will in your life, he will direct your path. Hear me when I say that this-is not an easy process and that there will be pain along the way. But take heart in the fact that I have met many like myself, who have healed from mental illness using the tools I have written about in this book.

To be sure, it is extremely difficult to help yourself when you aren't in your right mind and I pray that you find a fantastic advocate to help you on your path to healing. An advocate is someone who can keep notes for you, encourage you, help you chart symptoms, and make sense of all the information you'll gather along the way. Doing this on your own is daunting, but an advocate makes this process so much more achievable. Ultimately, our God is the God of healing and he wants a full and beautiful life for you. My heart is for you to know that you are OK and you are not going crazy. Crazy, to me, is someone who has no hope and no answers. That is not you. God has answers for you. There is a reason for the way you feel and most importantly, your condition can be healed. Like any physical ailment, I do believe that mental health and wellness starts in the gut. Eating a pure diet, exercising, praying every day, and having safe people in your life who love you and support you are all key to healing.

Avoid antidepressants and anti-anxiety medication if you can. These substances do not heal the real challenge; they simply cover it up. The real issue is that you are not getting the nutrients you need to help your mind function properly. There are some amazing forward-thinking doctors working in the field of mental health who are not using pharmaceuticals to simply mask the symptoms of nutrient deficiency or a compromised biochemistry. You will find more detailed information in the "Resources" section in the back of the book.

In my own journey, I could handle the physical aches and pains, but what really brought me to my knees was fearfulness, sadness, and irrational thoughts. There is hope for you and this can be cured.

BECOMING A BACKYARD FARMER

Eating this pure way often entices you to want to know more about where your food comes from. It can be time consuming to have to track down local producers. It is worth it, but I have found for my own schedule, that having a few egg chickens in my backyard is an easy way to supervise exactly what my chicken is eating. Having a small garden for veggies for dinner is a wonderful way to connect with your food. Letting friends know that you will take any leftover organic produce off their hands can result in a bounty of fruit and veggies, if you will come and pick them. Learning to cook new and exciting dishes that you might not otherwise eat can come of being willing to think outside the box and accept great food if its offered to you in the form of a surplus for another farmer. All it will cost you is your time to go pick them up!

Canning is another great way to preserve a harvest. I don't go crazy with this, but I do want access to healthy food all year long and I also want to do this on a budget. One thing to remember with canning is that heating food to a very high temperature can kill off many nutrients. Never can sauerkraut or other ferments as it destroys the enzymes and bacteria. however, when faced with a bumper crop of apples, canning can be woonderful. Right now, I have a small garden tower in my backyard that holds fifty plants. This has a worm composter in the middle, and it works great, giving me access to produce that is up off the ground to keep it from being eaten by my chickens or the local bunnies. Rethink how you see your food. We do raise meat chickens once or twice a year because it is a paltry ten-week commitment, very affordable, and fairly easy to do. At the end of the process, you absolutely know what went into that chicken. If you've ever tried to buy organic chicken at the store, you know how precious it is. For just a small amount of money and a gated puppy run, you can raise your own meat and ensure that you know where it comes from.

Egg chickens require very little effort and provide you with nutritious eggs, the likes of which don't even compare to grocery store eggs. If you've never had a fresh egg, you are missing out. Those hungry hens provide fertilizer for your grass and they eat the bugs. It's also relaxing to watch your chickens root around and scratch, as chickens do. I have found it to be a win-win.

Some of you might not be ready for this step and that's OK, too. This is only an option for those who want to progress a little deeper into this lifestyle. Currently, we live in a rental property and want to keep it nice so these small touches allow us to be connected to our food. I still support and get the bulk of what we eat from local ranches and farms, but I play some small part in my own food production and that can bring with it a huge sense of satisfaction.

PARTING THOUGHTS

"One of the biggest tragedies of human civilization is the precedents of chemical therapy over nutrition. It's a substitution of artificial therapy over nature, of poisons over food, in which we are feeding people poisons trying to correct the reactions of starvation."

-Dr. Royal Lee

I'd love to share so much more with you. I haven't included desserts or how to travel while eating this way and so many more tips and tricks, but that will have to wait for my next book. Look for that in a future book. What I have given you is a foundation. This is the best place to start when you are probably overwhelmed with the prospect of a big change in your life.

What I do know is this; food affects every aspect of our

lives. This is the sole pivot point on which your mental health, physical health, and energy rests. I hope you've realized that by now. Take some time and conduct an experiment of your own to watch people and what they eat. For the most part, you'll see that people who walk around with a soda pop in their hands don't look healthy, happy, and vibrant. In my experience, they look tired, unhappy, and overweight. Next, take a trip to your local health food store. No matter what you may think at first, these customers seem to be thinner, have lots of energy, and are smiling. Eating better produces better results.

I feel privileged that you have purchased this book and that you are contemplating change—even if it's a small change. No matter what, I encourage you to make one change. One change, followed by another change, followed by another change, can improve your life enormously. The

"Many little people, doing many little things, can change the world forever."
-German Proverb

Germans have a saying that goes like this:

Thank you so much for joining me on this journey. I am confident that you are on your way to vibrant, sustainable, abundant health for you and your family. Please do let me know how it goes.

Warmly.

RESOURCES & DEFINITIONS

RESOURCES

- My website: www.faithfoodhealing.com
- Wilderness Family Naturals: www.wildernessfamilynaturals.com.
- Frontier Organics: www.frontiercoop.com
- Low Energy Neurofeedback: www.ochslabs.com
- Alternative Mental Health Practitioners and Clinics: www.alternativetomeds.com, www.aadp.net
- The Weston A. Price organization: www.westonaprice.org
- Seafood: www.VitalChoice.com
- Amino Acid Therapy: www.everywomanover29.com
- Amino Acid Therapy Practitioner: Laurie Hammer, NT, Walker Chiropractic and Wellness, (515) 200-0020
- Nature Had It First: www.naturehaditfirst.com
- Natural Grocers Grocery Stores: www.naturalgrocers.com
- Drugless Practitioners of America: http://aadp.net/
- The Walsh Institute: http://www.walshinstitute.org/
- Alternative to Meds Center: https://www.alternativetomeds.com/
- The Nevada Clinic for Homeopathy: http://www.nevadaclinic.com/

DEFINITIONS

Pastured chicken: A chicken that is out in the grass, eating bugs and doing what chickens do. It is a myth that chickens will go outside and eat bugs on their own if they are fed lots of grain. They are lazy, too, so they have to be encouraged to go outside each day and forage. Don't confuse the term "pastured" with the term "cage-free." "Cage-free" are often chickens that have access to the outdoors (it could be a very small door that leads to a concrete and fenced in slab) but rarely go outside. You want eggs from pastured chickens and meat from pastured chickens.

"I bought a free-range chicken. You know, the kind that runs free and gets pampered like a family pet, right up until the day they kill it. It tasted surprised."

-Art Krug, Comedian

Pastured pork: Pigs that are raised out on pasture. Pork is the most abused animal in our food system. Never buy or eat pork unless you know where it came from. Large factory pork slaughterhouses provide horrific living conditions for pigs. Your meat should be as happy as it can be before it is processed and comes to your table.

Grass-fed and grass-finished beef: Beef cattle that are raised entirely on grass throughout their life up until the moment they are "processed". This definition can be deceiving. Don't be fooled by grocery store meat claiming to be grass-fed. There are no regulations or any standards for companies to use this term. If that beef cow has munched on hay during his life, he can be termed "grass-fed." This is why it is important to know your farmer. Please go and see for yourself how your animal lives and what it is eating.

GMO: The acronym for Genetically Modified Organism. This means someone in a lab coat with a degree in science has altered the genetic code of the plant. Most soy is GMO. So is most corn (unless labeled non-GMO), and varieties of tomatoes, sugarbeets (which is commonly used as the sugar source), as well as cotton. Cotton is important to note because of women's feminine products. Think about it—if you are using feminine products that carry pesticides that are designed to kill bacteria, good or bad, and you are putting them in sensitive places, that is not a good thing. Many varieties of veggies are GMO. GMO's have been linked to disease, autism, and food allergies. For more information on this subject, refer to the book Genetic Roulette: The Documented Health Risks of Genetically Engineered Foods by Jeffrey M. Smith or Youtube videos with Dr. Stephanie Seneff.

Amino Acids: Amino acids are organic compounds. Essential amino acids are essential for life and need to be obtained from food. The list of Essential amino acids includes valine, isoleucine, leucine, lysine, methionine, phenylalanine, threonine and tryptophan (and histidine for babies). Non-essential amino acids are still vital for life, but usually our body can make them without getting them through food. When we are ill or stressed, our body stops producing them and this can lead to deficiency and illness. These are vitally important to our health too so don't be misled by the label of non-essential. They are arginine, glutamine, tyrosine, cysteine, glycine, proline, serine and ornithine, alanine, asparagine and aspartate.

Neurofeedback and low-energy neurofeedback (LENS): LENS is a form of neurofeedback designed to retrain the brain when it has suffered trauma through a physical injury, emotional injury, or an illness.

Apple cider vinegar: This is a true fermented product. Many brands on the market today are not fermented, but instead are a product of food "additives." A couple of excellent brands of "living" fermented apple cider vinegar include Mother's or Bragg's brand. Real, living apple cider vinegar is essential to the recipes in this book.

Salt: As the recipes in this book convey, using real salt is a MUST. Real salt should always have a color. When your salt is colored, that means that it hasn't been bleached in any way and retains all of its mineral components. Most Americans never get to enjoy real salt. We're used to the refined, bleached and chemically processed salt that we have grown up with. Real salt has a distinctive taste and depending on where in the world it is farmed, has unique properties. Personally, I enjoy gray celtic sea salt or Redmond's salt from Utah. Redmond Salt has 60 trace minerals and a great taste too.

BIBLIOGRAPHY

Andrews, Ryan. All About Where Vitamin Supplements Come From. 2014. Retrieved from http://www.precisionnutrition.com/all-about-vitamin-supplements

Bland, Jeffrey, PhD. The Disease Delusion: Conquering the Causes of Chronic Illness for a Healthier, Longer, and Happier Life. New York. HarperCollins Books. 2014

Brockley, Annesse, Urdiales, Kristin. Autoimmune: The Cause and the Cure. Nature Had It First. Spearfish. 2013.

Butler, Carolyn. Hidden Hazards in Fruits and Veggies. Retrieved from http://www.washingtonpost.com/wp-dyn/content/article/2010/05/31/AR2010053101914.html

Fallon, Sally, Enig, Mary, PhD. Nourishing Traditions: The Cookbook that Challenges Politically Correct Nutrition and the Diet Dictocrats. Washington DC: New Trends Publishing, 2001.

Kressor, Chris. The high price of antibiotic use; can our guts ever recover? Retrieved from https://chriskresser.com/the-high-price-of-antibiotic-use-can-our-guts-ever-fully-recover/

Lite, Jordan. Vitamin D deficiency soars in the U.S., study says. Retrieved from http://www.scientificamerican.com/article/vitamin-d-deficiency-united-states/

Loux, Renee. Top 10 Reasons to Go Organic. Retrieved from http://www.prevention.com/food/healthy-eating-tips/top-reasons-choose-organic-foods

Mercola, Joseph, MD. If You Take Vitamin D You MUST Avoid This Serious Mistake. Retrieved from http://articles.mercola.com/sites/articles/archive/2012/02/23/oral-vitamin-d-mistake.aspx

Mercola, Joseph, MD. Why Did the Russians Ban an Appliance Found in 90% of American Homes? Retrieved from http://articles.mercola.com/sites/articles/archive/2010/05/18/microwave-hazards.aspx.2010

Myers, Amy, MD. 10 Signs You Have an Unhealthy Gut + How to Heal It. Retrieved from http://www.mindbodygreen.com/0-14510/10-signs-you-have-an-unhealthy-gut-how-to-heal-it.html

Perlmutter, David, MD. Grain Brain: The Surprising Truth about Wheat, Carbs, and Sugar—Your Brain's Silent Killers. New York. Little Brown. 2013.

Ross, Julia. The Mood Cure: The 4-Step Program to Take Charge of Your Emotions—Today. Penguin Books. London. 2002

Smith, Jeffrey, Seneff, Stephanie. The Health Dangers of Roundup Herbicide. Retrieved from https://www.youtube.com/watch?v=h_AHLDXF5aw. 2014.

Weil, Andrew, MD. Is Coconut Sugar a Healthier Sweetener? Retrieved from http://www.drweil.com/drw/u/QAA401323/Is-Coconut-Sugar-a-Healthier-Sweetener.html. 2016

80 percent of U.S. teens have bad diet. Retrieved from http://www.upi.com/Health_News/2013/04/07/80-percent-of-US-teens-have-a-bad-diet/13101365358161/. 2013
History of Kefir. Retrieved from http://kefir.biz/history.htm. 2002

The Chicken Soup Cure. Retrieved from http://nourishedkitchen.com/the-chicken-soup-cure/. 2009

The Dangers of Plastic. Retrieved from http://wellnessmama.com/23757/dangers-of-plastic/

Top 10 Reasons Bacon Is HEALTHY For You. Retrieved from https://bacontoday.com/top-10-reasons-bacon-is-actually-healthy-for-you/

SPECIAL THANKS

Enormous thanks to the following people. Without their support, ideas, love, and friendship as well as their cooking skills, editing skills, and amazing gifts, this book would not have been possible:

Roger Sherman, my sweet husband
Joy Duprey, my sister
Dorothy Distel, my mom
Bill Distel, my dad
Barbara Sherman, my mother-in-law
Brandee Knowles
Laurie Hammer, NMT
Dawn Shelstadt, my first raw milk farmer and a wealth of knowledge
Sheila Myers, a great friend
My cousin Keith for his recipe contributions.

The Colorado Springs Book Club Girls: A huge thanks for taking care of me for many years when I needed support and a shoulder to cry on.

Omaha Area GAPS Group: You are a continuous source of inspiration and an amazing example of determination to heal. I'm honored to call you friends.
My farmers, and ranchers, and to many who have taught me on my own journey of healing.

96496128R00096

Made in the USA
Columbia, SC
29 May 2018